MW00904937

GOLF FIT

The Only Guide You'll Need to Get You and Your Golf Game in Shape

GOLF FIT

The Only Guide You'll Need to Get You and Your Golf Game in Shape

Clay S. Harrow

Andrews and McMeel
A Universal Press Syndicate Company
Kansas City

Golf Fit: The Only Guide You'll Need to Get You and Your Golf Game in Shape
© 1997 by Clay S. Harrow. All rights reserved. Printed in the United States of
America. No part of this book may be used or reproduced in any manner what-
soever without written permission except in the case of reprints in the con-
text of reviews. For information, write Andrews and McMeel, a Universal Press
Syndicate Company, 4520 Main Street, Kansas City, Missouri 64111-7701.

Library of Congress Cataloging-in-Publication Data

Harrow, Clay S.
    Golf fit : the only guide you'll need to get you and your golf game in shape /
by Clay S. Harrow.
       p.   cm.
    ISBN 0-8362-2717-4 (pbk.)
    1. Golf—Training. 2. Physical fitness. I. Title.
GV979.T68H37   1997
796.352'3—dc20   96–43426
                                                     CIP

——————— **ATTENTION: SCHOOLS AND BUSINESS** ———————

Andrews and McMeel books are available at quantity discounts with
bulk purchase for educational, business, or sales promotional use.
For information, please write to: Special Sales Department, Andrews
and McMeel, 4520 Main Street, Kansas City, Missouri 64111-7701.

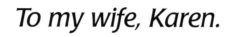

To my wife, Karen.

Contents

Foreword

Throughout the years, many people have sought my advice on how they could train specific muscles that had become sore or injured from participation in a particular sport. By chance, a large number of the complaints of injury and soreness came from golfers. These complaints included constant lower back pain, shoulder injuries and aches, and pain in the arms and legs. What surprised me the most about these complaints was the apparent source of the pain and injuries because, like many others, I had until then thought of golf as an inactive, physically unchallenging activity.

I gave these individuals my time and advice and showed them how to perform particular exercises to target the specific sore or injured muscles. By targeting the specific sore or injured muscles, I explained, they could strengthen and stretch the particular muscles and thereby decrease soreness, minimize risk of future injury, and improve their overall sport performance.

I noticed that many of the people who sought my advice and who did not previously exercise on a regular basis soon began to regularly perform the exercises I had given them and requested that I show them additional exercises to develop other muscles used in the particular sport in which they participated. This surprised me because these people had previously claimed that they lacked the available time to exercise on a regular basis. In addition, for many of those who sought my advice and who did participate in a general fitness program, I noticed that their general fitness programs soon became specific fitness programs designed to alleviate aches, pains, and strains from sport participation and to improve their sport performance.

These results were encouraging, but it seemed that the best use of this type of sport-specific training was to use it to train preventatively to avoid injuries and aches resulting from specific sporting activities before they occur and to increase the strength and flexibility of specific muscles in order to improve sport performance. Thus, what started out as a group of exercises given to people to train specific muscles that had become sore or injured from participation in a particular sport soon transformed into entire programs designed to minimize soreness and risk of injury and to improve performance in that sport. I had known that professional athletes had used sport-specific training to improve performance but had questioned its applicability to amateur athletes at much lower levels of ability and with less time and motivation for training.

The results were startling. Not only did these amateur athletes experience significant improvements in sport performance, in addition to less soreness and injury, but they also experienced greater energy and improved concentration during sport participation. Even better, they experienced increased motivation and enthusiasm for training because now they were training with a specific goal and purpose: better performance in a sport they enjoyed.

I began to speak with others about specific sports in which they participated, designed specific exercise programs to train the specific muscles used in that sport, and noticed the same results—improved performance, less soreness and injury, greater energy and concentration, and increased motivation for training. This proved to me firsthand the benefits of sport-specific training and, perhaps more important, that these benefits can be achieved by amateur athletes of all ages and levels of ability. I prefer to call this type of sport-specific training *sport performance training*, or simply *performance training*, because that term most accurately describes what it is—training to improve performance in a particular sport.

At the insistence of many of those who benefited from the exercises and programs I developed for them, as well as friends and family members who noticed my enthusiasm for performance training, I agreed to publish some of the exercises and routines I developed so that more amateur athletes can experience the benefits of performance training. *Golf Fit* is the first of such publications.

CHAPTER 1
About *Golf Fit*

If someone told you that you could significantly lower your golf score in the privacy of your own home, without picking up a golf club or hitting a golf ball, would you believe him? Probably not. Without additional private lessons, or spending hours on the practice range, hitting ball after ball? No way! Yet that is exactly what you can do, regardless of your age or level of play, by using the scientifically developed and proven flexibility and strength training exercises and routines described in this book, which were specifically designed to stretch and strengthen the specific muscles golfers use during a round of golf. To make matters even better, these same exercises and routines can also:

1. Minimize your risk of injury
2. Decrease your tendency to develop muscle aches and pains after golf
3. Increase your energy level
4. Improve your ability to concentrate
5. Increase your longevity and enjoyment of golf
6. Improve your overall strength, flexibility, and fitness

An improved golf game, and these other beneficial results, are achieved by performing the exercises and routines described in this book, which were developed by applying sport-specific performance training principles to the sport of golf.

About Sport-Specific Performance Training

It is no secret to professional athletes of all sports that performance in a particular sport can be significantly improved by increasing the strength and flexibility of the specific muscles used in that sport. In fact, many professional athletes reach a level of sport performance that can no longer be improved by continued practice of the particular sport movements and can only be improved by an overall increase in strength and flexibility of the specific muscles used in that sport. I refer to the performance of exercises and routines designed to strengthen and stretch specific muscles used in a particular sport in order to enhance performance in that sport as sport performance training or, more simply, *performance training*. The proven benefits of performance training can be achieved with equal success in any sport and by all participants, regardless of the individual's age or level of play. To date, however, performance training has been accepted and used almost exclusively by professional athletes.

Golf Fit presents performance training to amateur golfers in a manner that is easy to understand and can be incorporated into their lifestyles in order to allow them to benefit from performance training in the same way as professionals do, thus allowing them to improve their golfing ability, minimize muscle soreness and risk of injury, and increase their enjoyment of golf. I believe that *Golf Fit* is a breakthrough in applying performance training to golf for amateur athletes.

Golf Fit—Sport Performance Training for Golfers

As with professional athletes, one of the most critical factors limiting golf performance for many amateur golfers is their fitness level and, more specifically, the strength and range of motion (flexibility) of the specific muscles used in a round of golf. Simply because amateur golfers may have less available time or motivation for training than professional athletes—after all, amateur golfers must fit training and golf into otherwise busy schedules—doesn't mean that amateur golfers can't benefit from performance training. In fact, this is precisely the reason amateur golfers can benefit the most from performance training. By focusing on the specific muscles used in golf, performance training presents the most efficient way, in terms of time and energy, for amateur golfers to improve their golf performance through training. Further, performance training represents *fitness with a purpose*, and is thereby inherently more interesting and productive, and will result in better adherence to exercise schedules, particularly as schedules get busier and individuals have less time and motivation to devote to training.

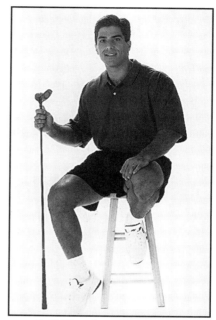

Golf Fit author Clay Harrow

If you haven't noticed by now, *Golf Fit* is not just another golf or fitness book. *Golf Fit* presents to amateur golfers a proven method of training for golf, i.e., performance training, previously enjoyed almost exclusively by professional golfers. The exercises and routines developed and described in *Golf Fit* were designed specifically for golfers. Unlike the exercises and routines found in most exercise programs, the *Golf Fit* exercises and routines do not focus on building larger muscles because larger muscles won't make you hit a golf ball any farther or closer to the pin. Rather, the *Golf Fit* exercises and routines focus on increasing the strength and flexibility of the specific muscles used in a golf swing, as well as other muscles used in a round of golf, based on the knowledge that improved golf performance, as well as other beneficial results, will directly result by increasing the strength and flexibility of these particular muscles.

The *Golf Fit* Advantage

Golf Fit provides the most efficient and productive way to improve golfing ability through fitness training and presents it in a manner that is easy to understand and incorporate into your lifestyle.

First, by targeting the specific golf muscles (i.e., those used in the golf swing, as well as other muscles used in a round of golf), *Golf Fit* contains the most efficient exercises and routines, in terms of time and energy, for the golf enthusiast. Each exercise in the *Golf Fit* routines is designed to train a specific golf muscle or group of muscles. Further, each exercise is designed to strengthen or stretch that specific golf muscle or group of muscles in a manner and through a range of motion that most closely resembles the way such muscles are used in a round of golf, thereby developing muscle memory and increasing the ability of that muscle to perform in the specific manner in which such muscle is used in a round of golf. General exercise programs may strengthen or stretch a specific muscle that, by chance, happens to be used in a round of golf, but such general exercise programs won't develop that muscle in a manner designed to improve its use in golf. Moreover, general exercise programs don't exercise all muscles used in golf, and they devote significant time and energy to muscles that won't improve golf performance. This is why *Golf Fit* will produce better results than any general exercise program and why *Golf Fit* presents the most effective and efficient exercises and routines for the amateur golfer.

Moreover, *Golf Fit* has been specifically developed with the amateur golfer in mind. Attention has been paid to providing alternative programs that can be incorporated into almost any busy schedule. *Golf Fit* provides the user with the ability to vary routines to fit within busier times and allow for varied workouts. These factors will increase adherence to the exercise program, thereby allowing for even faster and greater results.

Why Do I Need *Golf Fit*?

For years many people questioned the benefits of fitness training for golf. These people, whether professional or amateur golfers, golf spectators, researchers, or trainers, generally thought of golf as just a leisurely walk in the park or a pleasant way to spend some time on a weekend morning. What these people failed to realize is that a round of golf, while somewhat less aerobically demanding than other sports, requires a significant amount of physical activity and that much of the physical activity involves unnatural body movements performed in less than ideal conditions.

Walking or riding the golf course in itself requires substantial physical activity. The length of the average golf course is over seven thousand yards—*that's over four miles!* If someone told you that every weekend you would go out and walk over four miles, or ride over four miles in a golf cart, getting in and out over a hundred times, over a period of four hours or so, and that during that time you would also bend and pick up balls, tees, and flags over a hundred times, and take a hundred or so swings with a golf club (not to mention practice swings), would you undertake to perform this level of activity without feeling the need to engage in some type of physical training? Not likely. Yet that is exactly what most golfers do, week in and week out, year after year.

Now let's look at the golf swing itself, which for the average golfer is performed about one hundred times over the course of a round of golf (not counting practice swings or practice shots on the range). The average swing speed of an amateur golfer is almost ninety miles per hour, causing a pulling force of the golf club on the body of over one hundred pounds. On portions of a golf swing, parts of your body are actually moving in two directions at once, and the swing involves extreme shifts of weight from one side of the body to the other. Further, all of this occurs in an unnatural stance that itself places added strain and pressure on the shoulders, lower back, arms, and legs. And all this occurs in the perfect golf swing and with an ideal lie! A less than perfect swing (which is probably the case for most amateur golfers) taken on an uphill or downhill lie serves to multiply the undue strains and pressures on the body.

Even further, imagine all this occurring in less than ideal conditions—heat, humidity, or rain—throw in some frustration caused by some poor shots, and the result is both physical and mental fatigue providing ideal conditions for decreased physical performance, mental errors, and injury.

Understanding this, it is easy to see why proper training is beneficial, important, and even critical to good golf. Without proper training, these factors will inevitably take their toll on one's body, resulting in muscle soreness and injuries, decreased longevity, and, overall, less enjoyment of the game. This is particularly true as many golfers age and the adverse effects of these factors become even more pronounced, and if the individual leads an otherwise sedentary lifestyle.

Who Can Benefit from *Golf Fit*?

If you still need some convincing of the importance of performance training for golf, or if you question whether you, in particular, can benefit from *Golf Fit*, try answering a few of these questions:

- Do you consider yourself a slow starter on the golf course?

- Does it take you a few holes to get into your regular game?
- Are your scores on the first few holes generally higher than on later holes of equal difficulty?
- Are your scores on the front nine holes consistently higher than the back nine?

If your answer to any of these questions is yes, you suffer from inadequate warm-up and muscle conditioning, and you can benefit from _Golf Fit_.

Now, look at your swing in the mirror (or, better yet, on videotape):

- Is your swing any less than a natural flowing movement?
- Are there any hitches?
- Does your swing involve less than a full range of motion, from full backswing to full extension on the follow-through?
- Do you find that you must remind yourself to perform a full backswing or follow-through and make a deliberate effort to do so?
- Is your swing any shorter or less powerful than it once was?

If your answer to any of these questions is yes, you suffer from inadequate strength or range of motion of particular golf muscles, and you can benefit from _Golf Fit_.

On later holes:

- Do you tend to become more easily frustrated?
- Is your shot selection poorer?
- Do you have less patience or feel as if you are rushing to finish the round and get into the clubhouse?

If your answer to any of these questions is yes, you suffer from physical or mental fatigue during a round of golf, and you can benefit from *Golf Fit*.

Do you often:

- Experience muscle aches and pains the day after a round of golf?
- Feel as if you need a couple of days to recuperate between rounds of golf?
- Experience recurring injury to a particular muscle?

If your answer to any of these questions is yes, you suffer from inadequate muscle flexibility and conditioning, and you can benefit from *Golf Fit*.

By increasing the strength and flexibility of your golf muscles, *Golf Fit* can improve your golf performance and decrease the likelihood of your suffering from any of these problems. Despite the foregoing points, some individuals may still be skeptical about the benefits of performing specific exercises to improve your golf game. Perhaps this skepticism comes from seeing certain professional golfers who appear in less than ideal physical condition. For these skeptics, let me remind you that *Golf Fit* will not, in and of itself, make you a scratch golfer. As with any sport, one must incorporate both a strength and flexibility routine and practice of specific sport skills to achieve optimum performance. What *Golf Fit* will do, however, is make you a *better* golfer by increasing the strength and flexibility of your golf muscles. Remember that the relevant point of reference in evaluating the benefits to be gained from *Golf Fit* is your own golfing ability. Can there be any doubt that your golf game will improve if you have stronger and more flexible golf muscles?

Moreover, if you think you can't benefit from *Golf Fit* because you've never exercised before, you're exactly wrong! In fact, you are among the lucky ones because if you've never exercised before or do not currently participate in a regular exercise program, you can experience the quickest and most dramatic results from *Golf Fit*. *Golf Fit* takes you step by step through each exercise, explaining the proper way to perform each exercise, the muscle group or groups targeted by the exercise, as well as some common mistakes to avoid when performing each exercise, all in easy-to-understand terms and with photos. Further, *Golf Fit* tells you how to design a program specifically for you based on your current fitness level, time availability, and motivation and tells you how to chart your progress on each exercise and through each routine.

How *Golf Fit* Works

Understanding how *Golf Fit* works requires a brief description of how the human body works. The human body is a highly sensitive and proficient machine. It automatically and involuntarily seeks to attain a level of comfort and to avoid discomfort or pain, even discomfort or pain that we cannot experience consciously. When a particular movement is performed, the body automatically and involuntarily performs the movement in a manner consistent with these goals. For example, if a particular muscle that is involved in performing a proper golf swing is not strong or flexible enough to perform the movement through its entire range of motion, your body will automatically, involuntarily, and unconsciously compensate for the inadequacy of this muscle by using other muscles to compensate for the lack of strength of the proper muscle or by limiting the range of motion of the swing to compensate for the lack of flexibility of that muscle. The same is true if a movement involved in performing a proper golf swing causes pain from an injured or sore muscle, in which case the body automatically adjusts its movements to avoid this pain. The result in each case is a less than proper golf swing, using inappropriate muscles through a less than full range of motion.

13

This causes loss of power and accuracy and makes the individual more prone to injury. The swing is also less efficient, requiring more energy than a proper swing using the appropriate muscles through a full range of motion.

Often the cure sought for an improper swing caused by inadequate strength or flexibility of a particular golf muscle is for the golfer deliberately and consciously to try to compensate for the inadequacy in order to perform a swing that appears more correct. This is, at best, only a short-term fix, however, because the deliberate movement may use inappropriate muscles to compensate for a lack of strength in the proper golf muscle, or an increased range of motion may be achieved by performing improper movements undertaken to compensate for lack of flexibility of the proper golf muscle. In either case, the "corrected" swing is, at best, inefficient and unsafe. Further, the body will automatically and involuntarily revert to the improper, overcompensating movement as soon as your attention is diverted to another aspect of your swing. Deliberate and conscious efforts taken to cure an improper swing in this manner are merely attempts to treat the symptom, i.e., the improper golf swing, and in no way offer any lasting cure for the underlying problem, i.e., inadequate strength or flexibility of the relevant golf muscle. Further, deliberate and conscious efforts to achieve a proper golf swing cause, in many people, the overwhelming feeling that a proper golf swing requires them to concentrate on too many things at once.

One specific example of improper movements undertaken to compensate for lack of flexibility of the proper golf muscle occurs in many older golfers. As a result of growing older and inadequate flexibility training, many older golfers have significant limitations on the range of motion of their upper torso. The proper golf swing requires the upper body and shoulders to rotate almost twice as much as the hips. The limitation on upper body and shoulder rotation causes these golfers to overcompensate for their inadequate upper body and shoulder flexibility by adding an inappropriate degree of hip rotation. This results in a less than efficient golf swing, with less power and accuracy, and added strain on the lower back and hips resulting from overrotation, making them more prone to injury. *Golf Fit* will allow these golfers to increase the range of motion of the muscles of their upper body and shoulders, allowing their bodies to perform the proper degree of upper body and shoulder rotation and requiring less hip rotation, resulting in a better, more efficient golf swing and making them less prone to soreness and injury.

Another example of improper movements undertaken to compensate for lack of strength and flexibility of the proper golf muscles can be seen in many golfers who incorporate a hitch, or added movement, at the top portion of their backswing. These golfers suffer from a lack of flexibility necessary to enable them to perform a proper golf swing smoothly through a full range of motion, as well as a lack of strength necessary to maintain the golf club in its proper position throughout the swing. In an attempt to compensate for this inadequate muscle strength and flexibility, these golfers deliberately and consciously throw their club back at the top of their backswing, just before beginning their downswing. The result is a noticeable hitch in the golf swing, making it less efficient, with less power and accuracy, and placing added strain on the shoulders, hips, and legs by requiring an extension beyond their capable range of motion, making these muscles more prone to soreness and injury.

Take a look at the swing of professional golfers. Notice how it appears as a flowing, effortless movement, throughout a full range of motion? This is how a golf swing should look. It is only possible, however, if your golf muscles are strong and flexible enough to perform the swing through its full range of motion without the need to compensate for inadequate strength and flexibility in your golf muscles.

The proper way to correct an imperfect swing resulting from inadequate strength and flexibility of your golf muscles is to increase the strength and flexibility of your golf muscles. *Golf Fit* can help you accomplish this. Once this is accomplished, your body will no longer automatically seek to overcompensate for inadequate strength or flexibility, and a fuller, more naturally flowing golf swing is attainable.

Realistically speaking, because of physical limitations, age, or other reasons, many golfers will never develop that flowing, effortless swing professional golfers have. This doesn't mean, however, that these people can't develop a swing that more closely *resembles* the professional's effortless swing. Remember, in evaluating your performance, the relevant point of reference is yourself. By performing the exercises and routines in *Golf Fit*, you can strengthen and stretch your golf muscles, thereby increasing the range of motion your body will automatically allow in your golf swing. You can decrease your body's tendency to overcompensate for inadequate strength and flexibility of your golf muscles by simply increasing the strength and flexibility of your golf muscles. The results may be somewhat less than the effortless swing of the professional, but you will be closer to achieving such a swing than you would have been without *Golf Fit*, and, perhaps more important, your swing will be safer, and you will be less prone to muscle soreness and injury.

The Benefits of *Golf Fit*

Some of the benefits that can achieved by performance of the *Golf Fit* exercises and routines are discussed briefly below:

Minimized Risk of Injury

I can imagine nothing more frustrating to a golfer than being forced to sit out a round of golf on a beautiful spring day because of an injury. Sure, you could sit home and watch the pros play on television, but this certainly isn't the preferred way to spend the day.

By properly conditioning your golf muscles through performance of the *Golf Fit* exercises and routines, your golf muscles will be stronger and in better condition to withstand the strains and pressures applied on them by the necessary movements required in a round of golf. This will make these muscles less prone to injury. Further, better-conditioned muscles will improve muscular endurance, resulting in less physical and mental fatigue during golf play. Physical and mental fatigue are prime factors leading to injury, and by decreasing these factors you will minimize your risk of injury. Moreover, by adopting and performing the Golf Fit Warm-Up Routine as part of your regular golfing procedure, your risk of injury will be significantly reduced.

Decreased Muscle Aches and Pains after Golf

Muscle aches and pains occurring twenty-four to forty-eight hours after golfing are the result of using the sore muscles in a manner to which they are not otherwise accustomed to being used. By performing the *Golf Fit* exercises and routines, your muscles will be accustomed to use in the precise manner in which they are used during a round of golf, resulting in less tendency to develop muscle aches and pains after golf play.

Increased Energy and Improved Concentration

As your muscles grow tired and sore during a round of golf, the natural result is both physical and mental fatigue which causes a decrease in your ability to focus and concentrate. Decreased concentration, in turn, causes physical and mental errors. By using the *Golf Fit* exercises and routines, you will improve your muscular endurance, thereby increasing your ability to concentrate, particularly on later holes, resulting in less tendency to make physical and mental errors and a better ability to focus on proper shot selection and hitting the golf ball. In addition, by properly conditioning the golf muscles, your swing will be using the proper muscles through their full range of motion, resulting in a more natural and efficient golf swing, which requires less energy to perform. The energy saved on each swing will be available on later holes.

Increased Longevity and Enjoyment

By properly conditioning your golf muscles through performance of the *Golf Fit* exercises and routines, these muscles will be stronger and in better condition to withstand the strains and pressures applied on them by the necessary movements required in a round of golf. This will decrease the natural tendency of the body to weaken and limit the range of motion of your muscles as you age. The result will be the ability to participate in golf longer and without the natural decrease in ability that would otherwise occur with age. This, together with the ability to play with less pain and injury, will certainly increase your enjoyment of the game of golf.

Improved Muscle Feel

Muscle feel is the term used to describe one's ability to sense the particular muscles of the body and to actually feel their use in particular movements. By performing the *Golf Fit* exercises and routines, you will become more aware of the particular muscles and how they are used in a proper golf swing, and you will develop a better feel for each golf muscle. This will enable you to better sense improper movements of specific muscles and correct such movements and also make you better able to correctly perform specific movements suggested to improve your golf swing.

Increased Level of Confidence

All golfers know the importance of confidence in golf. Knowing that your swing is more efficient, powerful, and accurate, and that you will have more energy and concentration throughout the round, will most certainly increase your overall confidence in your golfing ability.

Increased Strength, Flexibility and Overall Fitness

Performance of the *Golf Fit* exercises and routines will increase your muscular strength and flexibility as well as your overall fitness level and make you healthier and in better shape to perform everyday activities other than golf.

Better Golf

Less injury and pain, increased longevity and enjoyment, increased energy and improved concentration, greater confidence, and a safer, more efficient, powerful, and accurate golf swing—these are the principal factors leading to a better golf game.

How the *Golf Fit* Exercises and Routines Were Developed

The *Golf Fit* exercises and routines were developed through careful analysis of the golf swing and the muscle groups used throughout it. First, we broke down the golf swing into its component parts (i.e., address/stance, shoulder turn, hip turn, knee action, head and chin rotation, weight shift) and identified the specific muscle groups used during each component of the movement. Then we developed both strength and flexibility exercises for each of these muscle groups. The exercises were developed to increase the strength and flexibility of each muscle group in a way that closely resembles the manner in which each muscle group is used in the golf swing. In other words, the *Golf Fit* exercises were developed to exercise the particular muscle group in the position and throughout the range of motion that the muscle group is used in the golf swing. We also identified other muscle groups used in a round of golf (for example, those muscle groups used getting in and out of a golf cart, walking, and bending) and added exercises to strengthen and stretch them because strain and fatigue on these muscle groups will adversely effect your golf swing, concentration, and enjoyment, particularly on later holes.

The muscle groups we've identified and targeted and a brief description of their use in a round of golf are summarized in Table 1. As is evident from the table, each particular movement in the golf swing involves the use and coordination of more than one muscle or group of muscles to perform the movement properly. Further, larger movements in the golf swing, such as the rotation of the trunk, require the use and coordination of most major muscles of your body.

TABLE 1. Major Muscle Groups and Their Use in Golf

MAJOR MUSCLE GROUP	USE IN GOLF
Neck	The neck muscles are responsible for maintaining the proper head position at address, as well as for rotating the head throughout the golf swing.
Shoulders	The shoulder muscles are responsible for rotating the shoulders throughout the golf swing, as well as for lifting the golf club and carrying the arms throughout the golf swing, withstanding extreme pulling forces of the golf club during the swing, and creating and maintaining proper swing speed and speed of the club at impact.

MAJOR MUSCLE GROUP	USE IN GOLF
Chest	The chest muscles are involved in carrying and controlling the arms in front of the body during the golf swing, rotating the trunk, generating power, and maintaining proper swing speed and speed of the club at impact.
Upper Back	The upper back muscles are involved in rotating the trunk, lifting the golf club, and carrying the arms throughout the golf swing.
Lower Back	The lower back muscles are involved in rotating the trunk and maintaining the proper position at address and throughout the golf swing. The lower back muscles are particularly vulnerable to injury.
Hips	The hips are responsible for rotating the trunk, initiating the downswing, creating and maintaining proper swing speed, and creating power at impact.
Upper Legs	The hamstring (rear) and quadricep (front) muscles of the upper legs are responsible for generating a substantial portion of the power in the golf swing, rotating the trunk, withstanding the twisting forces of the upper body, and maintaining proper position and balance throughout the swing.

Major Muscle Group	Use in Golf
Abdominals	The abdominal muscles are responsible for rotating the trunk, maintaining proper position at address, and stabilizing the vulnerable muscles of the lower back.
Lower Legs	The calf muscles of the lower leg are responsible for maintaining proper balance throughout the golf swing and maintaining proper foot position at address and throughout the backswing and follow-through.
Upper Arms	The bicep (front) and tricep (rear) muscles of the upper arms are responsible for controlling and maintaining proper arm and club position throughout the golf swing; rotating, bending, and extending the arms; and generating club speed at impact.
Lower Arms	The muscles of the wrists and forearms are responsible for maintaining proper grip and controlling the proper position of the club throughout the entire golf swing and at impact.

Sticktoitiveness—The Key to Results

As with any general exercise program, sticktoitiveness (i.e., adherence to a regular program) is paramount. Improved strength and flexibility occur gradually over time and are achieved most successfully by regularly performing a properly designed program of exercises. Recent studies have identified several factors that increase the likelihood that an individual will adhere to a regular training program. These factors include the variability of the routine, the time commitment involved, the ease with which the routine can be incorporated into an individual's lifestyle, and the equipment needs of the training program. *Golf Fit* was developed with each of these factors in mind in order to make it easy for you to develop a proper training program and stick to it.

First, by focusing primarily on the particular muscles used in golf and choosing only those exercises essential to increasing the strength and range of motion of these muscles, *Golf Fit* is the most efficient set of exercises and routines, in terms of time and energy, for the golf enthusiast. Further, by grouping the various exercises into separate routines, the individual can mix and match the separate routines in order to tailor a program to meet his or her particular goals and fit within any particular individual constraints (e.g., time or motivation). *Golf Fit* can be used by golfers with a wide range of goals, including the desire to increase the strength and flexibility of their golf muscles during the off season, immediately prior to the start of the golf season, before embarking on a golf vacation, between golf outings during the golf season, or before returning to golf after a layoff or injury. Finally, with the exception of the *Golf Fit* advanced strength training exercises that require the use of small hand weights, all of the *Golf Fit* exercises were developed to be performed without the need for additional equipment or extraneous devices, and the amount of time spent moving from one exercise to the next has been minimized by efficient ordering of exercises.

23

How Do I Get Started?

Believe it or not, you've already taken your first step toward improving your golf game by picking up this book and recognizing what professional golfers know to be true but many amateur golfers simply refuse to believe: strength and flexibility performance training will improve golf performance. The next step is to make a commitment to improving your golf game and overall fitness level by choosing and performing the appropriate *Golf Fit* performance training program for you.

How to Use This Book

The *Golf Fit* exercises and routines were developed with the amateur golfer in mind and were designed to allow amateur golfers to develop and adopt a particular performance training program that will most appropriately meet their goals and fit within their schedules. In this regard, the particular *Golf Fit* strength and flexibility exercises are grouped into four component groups, referred to as *routines,* based on the primary purpose of performing that exercise. The four *Golf Fit* routines are the Golf Fit Warm-Up Routine, the Golf Fit Flexibility Training Routine *(Golf Flex)*, the Golf Fit Strength Training Routine *(Golf Strong)*, and the Golf Fit Short Routine. Each of these routines can be used as an entire program or as part of a longer program created by grouping together two or more separate routines, depending upon the individual's particular needs and limitations. Each of the four *Golf Fit* routines is described briefly under the following heading, The *Golf Fit* routines, together with the approximate amount of time it should take to perform the exercises involved. A more detailed description of each routine can be found under its separate chapter heading later in the book. Complete exercise programs comprised of groupings of the routines are described under the heading Recommended Training Programs.

The Golf Fit Routines

The Golf Fit Warm-Up Routine.

The Golf Fit Warm-Up Routine is composed of six movements designed to warm up the specific muscles used in a round of golf. It is designed to be used before practice shots on the range as well as before a round of golf. Further, because the *Golf Fit* strength and flexibility routines utilize the same muscles used in a round of golf, the Golf Fit Warm-Up Routine is also designed to be used as a warm-up before performance of these routines. The approximate time needed for performance of the Golf Fit Warm-Up Routine is eight minutes.

Golf Flex—The Golf Fit Flexibility Training Routine.

The Golf Fit Flexibility Training Routine, which we call *Golf Flex*, is specifically designed to lengthen and increase the range of motion of those muscles used in a golf swing and during a round of golf. It is composed of twelve stretching exercises, each aimed to stretch a particular golf muscle or group of muscles. The approximate time needed for performance of the Golf Fit Flexibility Training Routine is ten minutes.

Golf Strong—The Golf Fit Strength Training Routine.

The Golf Fit Strength Training Routine, which we call *Golf Strong*, is specifically designed to increase the strength of those muscles used in a golf swing and during a round of golf. It is composed of twelve strength training exercises, each aimed to strengthen and develop a particular golf muscle or group of muscles. The approximate time needed for performance of the Golf Fit Strength Training Routine is fifteen minutes.

For each of the basic *Golf Strong* exercises, we have included an advanced way of performing that particular exercise in order to allow for a progressive level of training, if desired, after a period of continued performance of the basic *Golf Strong* exercises. Some of the advanced exercises require the use of small hand weights in order to increase the resistance offered by the basic movements.

The Golf Fit Short Routine.

Through use of compound movements, the Golf Fit Short Routine is designed to work each of the major golf muscle groups in the shortest amount of time using the fewest number of total exercises. While somewhat less comprehensive than the *Golf Flex* and *Golf Strong* routines, this routine provides an alternative for those individuals who have a very limited amount of time to devote to training their golf muscles but still wish to experience the benefits offered to golfers by performance training, as well as those individuals who usually perform the longer routines but, on a particular day, may have a limited amount of time or prefer a shorter workout. It is composed of six compound exercises. The approximate time needed for performance of the Golf Fit Short Routine is eight minutes.

Recommended Training Programs

We have grouped together some of the *Golf Fit* routines described briefly above, and in more detail later in the book, into certain more complete training programs designed for individuals with particular goals and time availability. These suggested programs are described below.

The Golf Fit Full-Flexibility Training Program.

The Golf Fit Full-Flexibility Training Program is designed for those individuals seeking primarily to increase the flexibility and range of motion of their golf muscles. It consists of performing the Golf Fit Warm-Up Routine once, followed by performance of the Golf Fit Flexibility Training Routine twice. On the second time performing the Golf Fit Flexibility Training Routine, attention should be paid to stretching the particular muscles a bit farther than had been done the first time and holding the stretched position a bit longer. This program provides a complete training program for stretching the golf muscles to improve your golf game. The approximate time needed for performance of the Golf Fit Full-Flexibility Training Program is thirty minutes.

The Golf Fit Full-Strength Training Program.

The Golf Fit Full-Strength Training Program is designed for those individuals seeking primarily to increase the strength of their golf muscles. It consists of performing the Golf Fit Warm-Up Routine once, followed by performance of the Golf Fit Strength Training Routine twice. This program provides a complete training program for strengthening the golf muscles to improve your golf game. The approximate time needed for performance of the Golf Fit Full-Strength Training Program is forty minutes.

The Golf Fit Flexibility and Strength Training Program.

The Golf Fit Flexibility and Strength Training Program is designed for those individuals seeking to increase both the flexibility and strength of their golf muscles. It consists of performing the Golf Fit Warm-Up Routine once, followed by performance of the Golf Fit Flexibility Training Routine and the Golf Fit Strength Training Routine. This program provides a complete and balanced training program for both stretching and strengthening the golf muscles to improve your golf game. The approximate time needed for performance of the Golf Fit Flexibility and Strength Training Program is thirty-five minutes.

The Golf Fit Advanced Strength Training Program.

The Golf Fit Advanced Strength Training Program is designed for those individuals seeking primarily to increase the strength of their golf muscles and who are looking for a more progressive program than is offered by the Golf Fit Full-Strength Training Program. It consists of performing the Golf Fit Warm-Up Routine once, followed by performance of the Golf Fit Strength Training Routine twice using the advanced exercises. This program provides the most aggressive training program for strengthening the golf muscles to improve your golf game. It is designed for those who have been performing the Golf Fit Full-Strength Training Program regularly and are seeking a more progressive program or individuals who have been previously involved in strength training. The approximate time needed for performance of the Golf Fit Advanced Strength Training Program is forty minutes.

The Golf Fit Advanced Flexibility and Strength Training Program.

The Golf Fit Advanced Flexibility and Strength Training Program is designed for those individuals seeking the most comprehensive and aggressive way to increase the flexibility and range of motion of their golf muscles as well as the strength of their golf muscles. It consists of performing the Golf Fit Warm-Up Routine once, followed by performance of the Golf Fit Flexibility Training Routine twice, followed by performance of the Golf Fit Strength Training Routine twice. As the most comprehensive of the suggested training programs, it is also the most time consuming. The approximate time needed for performance of the Golf Fit Advanced Flexibility and Strength Training Program is sixty minutes.

The Golf Fit Short Training Program.

The Golf Fit Short Training Program is designed for those individuals seeking to increase the flexibility and strength of their golf muscles but who do not have the necessary time or motivation (either regularly or on a particular day) to perform any of the other suggested training programs. It consists of performing the Golf Fit Warm-Up Routine once, followed by performance of the Golf Fit Short Routine. The approximate time needed for performance of the Golf Fit Short Training Program is fifteen minutes.

Choosing a Program That's Right for You

Before choosing one of the suggested training programs described above or developing one of your own programs by grouping together the *Golf Fit* routines, we suggest that you realistically evaluate the time and energy you have to devote to a training program as well as your current fitness level. The reason for this is the importance in choosing or developing a program that you can and *will* fit within your lifestyle. If you choose or develop a program that takes longer than you realistically have available to exercise, or is simply too difficult for you to maintain at your current fitness level, you will likely discontinue exercise after a short period of time. Remember, exercise is not a competitive activity but merely a means to an end, i.e., better fitness and better golf, which is achieved gradually by continued performance of the routines and programs. Start slowly, and avoid any impulse to choose or develop a program that is too time consuming or strenuous for you. If you should choose a program that you find you cannot maintain, reevaluate your available time and energy and your current fitness level and choose or develop a program that is more appropriate for you. The most productive program for you is not necessarily the most comprehensive program that you can make it through once but rather the program that you can and will maintain over a period of time. A ten-minute program performed regularly and consistently is infinitely more beneficial than a longer routine performed occasionally.

Recommended Training Schedules

It is recommended that you initially perform whichever program you choose at least three times per week, with at least one but not more than two days' rest between sessions. After you have reached an initial level of fitness, you may wish to perform the routines more frequently or alternate between routines performed on consecutive days. In addition to your regular training schedule, it is also recommended that you perform the Golf Fit Warm-Up Routine prior to golf practice or play. Further, if you experience any muscle soreness or aches on a day following golf play or exercise, you may wish to perform the Golf Fit Flexibility Training Routine to help alleviate the soreness or aches.

Charting Your Progress

We suggest that you keep a detailed log of the performance of your exercise program, noting the date and time performed, the particular exercises performed, the length of time it took to perform the program, and the ease or difficulty of performance of each exercise and the overall program, as well as any subjective factors that may have influenced your performance, including layoff, diet, lack of sleep, motivation, and stress. Keeping a detailed log provides you with necessary feedback and is the best way to keep track of your progress, continually evaluate your current program, and make necessary modifications to your program.

Appendix C contains a recommended Golf Fit Training Log, which you may wish to use to chart your progress in performing the *Golf Fit* routines, as well as a sample filled-in log illustrating the proper manner in which to keep your training log. Feel free to copy these forms or modify them to meet your particular needs.

One Final Note Before Proceeding

As with any exercise program, always use common sense. Do not begin any exercise program without first consulting your physician and obtaining his or her consent. If at any time while exercising you experience nausea, dizziness, light-headedness, shortness of breath, or other signs of discomfort, stop exercising immediately and consult your physician as to the appropriate manner in which to proceed.

CHAPTER 2
The Golf Fit Warm-Up Routine

About the Golf Fit Warm-Up Routine

I can't tell you how many times I've walked onto a golf course or practice range and seen a golfer take a club out of the bag and step up to the ball, then back away from the ball and begin to swing the club haphazardly overhead, or bend from side to side for several seconds, or perform some other haphazard and potentially dangerous movements in an effort to warm up. Sound familiar? I've seen it hundreds of times, and I'm sure you have, too. It may even be you. Needless to say, this is not an adequate or at all effective warm-up, and it can be dangerous. The only thing more disturbing than the likelihood of these people injuring themselves by performing these movements is the likelihood of them injuring bystanders. I have, on more than one occasion, witnessed clubs fly out of the hands of golfers performing some of these "warm-up routines." My advice to you when you see an individual engaging in this sort of activity is to get out of his way!

The importance of adopting a proper warm-up routine and performing this routine each time you play, practice, or train cannot be overstated. You wouldn't expect a trainer to allow a prize racehorse to walk out of the stable and run the Kentucky Derby. We shouldn't treat our bodies with any less care and respect. Proper warm-up is the single most important thing you can do to minimize the risk of injury in any physical activity, including golf. If you take any one piece of advice from this book, let it be the importance of performing a proper warm-up each and every time you practice or play.

A proper warm-up serves to increase your overall body temperature, and also the temperature of specific muscles and other tissues. This improves muscle elasticity, enabling the muscles to bend and stretch more easily, which makes them more accommodating to extreme physical movements such as the golf swing, less prone to injury, and more able to perform at their optimal level. A proper warm-up also increases the heart rate, blood pressure and blood circulation, and oxygen supply throughout the body, places the entire body in a more ready state to perform physical activity, and reduces the potential for fatigue.

Inadequate warm-up is the primary reason many golfers complain of being slow starters, and that it takes them a few holes to get into their regular game. What these golfers are actually doing is using the first few holes of their golf game as their warm-up. Needless to say, this provides an inadequate warm-up, doesn't reduce the risk of injury, and results in higher scores.

Adopting a regular and consistent warm-up routine will also help psychologically by placing you in a more ready mental state for golf play. We've all seen golfers who adhere to a strict routine of movements each time they hit a tee shot. By performing this same strict routine each time, they have conditioned their body to be ready to perform a tee shot each time it recognizes that the preshot routine is performed. Adopting a proper warm-up routine and performing it each and every time you practice or play will work in much the same way. It will tell your body that golf will follow, and your body will respond automatically by placing itself in a more ready state. In addition, regular performance of a warm-up routine allows you to free your mind for several moments prior to play, resulting in a more relaxed and ready state, both physically and mentally.

In addition to the desire to play well, you should also seek to play smart. Playing smart requires incorporating a proper warm-up routine into your regular schedule. I understand fully the impulse of golfers to get out there and begin playing as soon as they get to the golf course. To play smart, however, you must try to control this urge long enough to perform a full and proper warm-up. The Golf Fit Warm-Up Routine contains six exercises designed to warm up your entire body. Furthermore, it was designed to do so in the least amount of time, through use of compound movements. The entire Golf Fit Warm-Up Routine should take no longer than eight minutes. Considering that the average round of golf takes four hours or so, eight minutes seems like a small sacrifice to make to minimize risk of injury and allow for safer and better play.

To insure that you perform the Golf Fit Warm-Up Routine before each and every time you practice or play, we suggest that you incorporate the Golf Fit Warm-Up Routine at the same point each time in your overall preplay routine. For example, you could perform the warm-up immediately after putting on your golf shoes, as soon as you step out of the clubhouse, just after signing in, or after getting your bucket of range balls. By performing the warm-up routine at the same time in your preplay routine, you will insure that the warm-up becomes a regular part of your pre-play activity and that you actually perform the warm-up routine each and every time you practice or play.

Each of the exercises in the Golf Fit Warm-Up Routine was designed to be performed while holding the golf club because holding the club while performing a warm-up will further increase the warm-up's effectiveness in preparing you psychologically for golf play. If you are performing the Golf Fit Warm-Up Routine at home or if you simply don't want to hold the club while warming up, you can perform each of these exercises just as effectively using a straight object such as a broomstick or without any object by simply holding your hands in the position they would be in if you were holding a club, e.g., on your shoulders if the exercise calls for holding the club behind your neck.

For your convenience, a chart containing each of the Golf Fit

Warm-Up Routine exercises is included as Appendix B. You can keep this chart in your golf bag or locker or carry it with you to the golf course or practice range to make sure you don't forget any of the Golf Fit Warm-Up Routine exercises.

For those of you who, in spite of the foregoing, will still avoid performing the Golf Fit Warm-Up Routine, let me make one last-ditch effort to get you to perform some warm-up activity. If you feel the Golf Fit Warm-Up Routine requires too much time, energy, commitment, motivation, or whatever and you know that you just won't perform the entire routine each and every time you practice or play, try to modify the routine to create a routine you will perform. In modifying the Golf Fit Warm-Up Routine, we suggest that you do not skip any of the exercises. Remember, the Golf Fit Warm-Up Routine was carefully designed to warm up *all* the major muscle groups used in golf. Instead, you can modify the routine by reducing the number of repetitions of each exercise. While such a modification will render the warm-up somewhat less effective than performance of the entire Golf Fit Warm-Up Routine, it will be infinitely more beneficial than performing no warm-up routine at all.

For each Golf Fit Warm-Up Routine exercise, we have described the proper starting position and the movement involved in detail and with photos. We have also listed certain points to focus on when performing the movement and the approximate time it should take to perform the movement.

The Golf Fit Warm-Up Routine—List of Exercises

Golf Fit Warm-Up Routine EXERCISE ONE: Knee Bends

Golf Fit Warm-Up Routine EXERCISE TWO: Bent Trunk Twists

Golf Fit Warm-Up Routine EXERCISE THREE: Overhead Side Bends

Golf Fit Warm-Up Routine EXERCISE FOUR: Good Mornings

Golf Fit Warm-Up Routine EXERCISE FIVE: Combination Presses

Golf Fit Warm-Up Routine EXERCISE SIX: Toe Raises

The Golf Fit Warm-Up Routine—In Detail

Golf Fit Warm-Up Routine *Exercise One: Knee Bends*

Starting Position:

Standing straight, feet shoulder-width apart, knees slightly bent, and toes pointed slightly outward. Place a club on your shoulders, behind your neck, and hold on to the club with each hand. (See Step 1.)

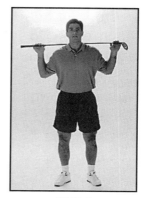

STEP 1

Description of Movement:

Slowly lower your body as far as you comfortably can, but not lower than parallel to the floor. Allow your heels to rise slightly off the floor as you lower your body. (See Step 2.) Pause at the bottom of the movement. Slowly raise your body to the original starting position. Pause at the top of the movement.

Focus On:

Slowly lowering and raising your body to a count of three and holding each pause for a count of one.

Keeping your back straight and your head up throughout the entire movement; avoiding leaning forward during the movement.

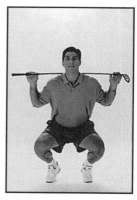

STEP 2

Keeping your knees and thighs from moving inward during the movement.

Number of Repetitions:

Perform this movement for twelve repetitions.

Approximate Time: 1 minute 30 seconds.

Golf Fit Warm-Up Routine *Exercise Two:*
Bent Trunk Twists

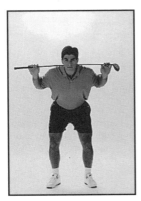

STEP 1

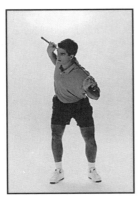

STEP 2

Starting Position:

Standing straight, feet shoulder-width apart, knees slightly bent, and toes pointed slightly outward. Place a club on your shoulders, behind your neck, and hold on to the club with each hand. Bend slightly at the waist, about one third of the way toward being parallel to the floor. (See Step 1.)

Description of Movement:

Slowly twist your upper body to one side as far as you comfortably can by moving your right shoulder toward the midpoint of your body. (See Step 2.) Pause at the end of the twist. Slowly twist your upper body to the opposite side as far as you comfortably can by moving your left shoulder toward the midpoint of your body. Pause at the end of the twist.

Focus On:

Slowly twisting your upper body to each side to a count of three and holding each pause for a count of one. Keeping your back straight and your head up throughout the entire movement.

Number of Repetitions:

Perform this movement for twelve repetitions.

Approximate Time: 1 minute 30 seconds.

Golf Fit Warm-Up Routine *Exercise Three: Overhead Side Bends*

Starting Position:

Standing straight, feet shoulder-width apart, knees slightly bent, and toes pointed slightly outward. Hold a club with both hands, slightly more than shoulder-width apart, and arms outstretched overhead. (See Step 1.)

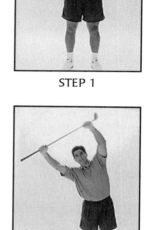

STEP 1

Description of Movement:

Slowly lean your upper body to one side as far as you comfortably can. (See Step 2.) Pause. Slowly return to the starting position. Pause. Slowly lean your upper body to the opposite side as far as you comfortably can. Pause. Slowly return to the starting position.

Focus On:

Slowly leaning your upper body to each side to a count of three and holding each pause for a count of one.

Keeping your back straight and your head up throughout the entire movement.

STEP 2

Keeping your upper body vertical during the entire movement; avoiding leaning forward or backward.

Number of Repetitions:

Perform this movement for six repetitions.

Approximate Time: 1 minute.

Golf Fit Warm-Up Routine *Exercise Four: Good Mornings*

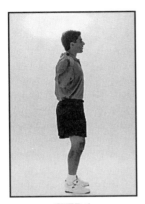

STEP 1

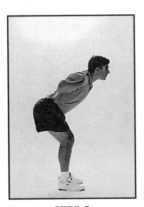

STEP 2

Starting Position:

Standing straight, feet shoulder-width apart, knees slightly bent, and toes pointed slightly outward. Place a club on your shoulders, behind your neck, and hold on to the club with each hand. (See Step 1.)

Description of Movement:

Keeping your back straight and head up, slowly bend forward at the waist as far as you comfortably can. (See Step 2.) Pause. Slowly raise your body to the starting position.

Focus On:

Slowly bending and raising your upper body to a count of three and holding each pause for a count of one.

Keeping your back straight and your head up throughout the entire movement.

Number of Repetitions:

Perform this movement for six repetitions.

Approximate Time: 1 minute.

Golf Fit Warm-Up Routine *Exercise Five: Combination Presses*

Starting Position:

Standing straight, feet shoulder-width apart, knees slightly bent, and toes pointed slightly outward. Hold a club with both hands, slightly more than shoulder-width apart, and arms extended downward. (See Step 1.)

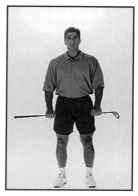

STEP 1

Description of Movement:

Slowly pull the club up to your chest. (See Step 2.) Pause. Slowly extend your arms forward. (See Step 3.) Pause. Slowly pull your arms back in to your chest. Pause. Slowly extend your arms overhead. (See Step 4.) Pause. Slowly pull your arms back down to your chest. Pause. Slowly extend your arms forward again. Pause. Slowly pull your arms back in to your chest. Pause. Slowly lower your arms to their original downward position.

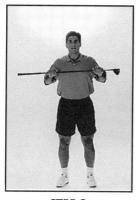

STEP 2

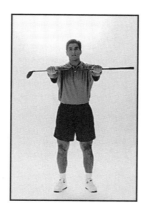

STEP 3

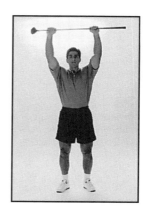

STEP 4

Focus On:

Slowly lifting, pulling, and extending the club on each movement. Keeping your back straight and your head up throughout the entire movement.

Number of Repetitions:

Perform this movement for six repetitions.

Approximate Time: 2 minutes.

Golf Fit Warm-Up Routine *Exercise Six: Toe Raises*

Starting Position:

Standing straight, feet shoulder-width apart, knees slightly bent, and toes pointed slightly outward. Hold a club with both hands, slightly more than shoulder-width apart, and arms extended downward. (See Step 1.)

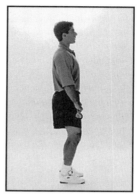

STEP 1

Description of Movement:

Slowly raise yourself up onto the balls of your feet as far as you comfortably can. (See Step 2.) Pause. Slowly lower yourself to the original starting position.

Focus On:

Slowly raising and lowering yourself each time to a count of three and holding each pause for a count of one.

Keeping your back straight and your head up throughout the entire movement.

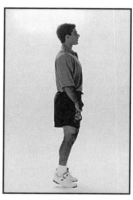

STEP 2

Number of Repetitions:

Perform this movement for twelve repetitions.

Approximate Time: 1 minute.

43

CHAPTER 3
Golf Flex –The Golf Fit
Flexibility Training Routine

About *Golf Flex*

In order to have a proper, safe, and efficient golf swing, you must have the necessary flexibility in your golf muscles to allow your body to perform the swing through the entire range of motion, from full backswing to extended follow-through. If your muscles lack this flexibility, whether because of injury, lack of use, or shortening caused by age, your body will be unable to perform a proper golf swing. The result is a less efficient, less powerful, and less accurate swing that requires more energy to perform and muscles that are more prone to injury, soreness, and fatigue.

The only way to increase the flexibility of your golf muscles is to perform stretching exercises designed to increase the range of motion of the necessary muscles. *Golf Flex* is designed to stretch all your golf muscles in a manner and through a range of motion that closely resembles the way such muscles are used in golf and to do so in the shortest amount of time. It is the most efficient and effective way to increase the flexibility and range of motion of your golf muscles and achieve a more powerful, efficient, and safer golf swing.

The *Golf Flex* routine consists of twelve stretching movements and should take approximately ten minutes to perform. While performing each of the *Golf Flex* exercises, remember to

- Perform each movement in a slow and controlled manner.
- Avoid quick or jerky movements.
- Never bounce while stretching. Bouncing causes the muscles to shorten and could cause injury.
- Breathe slowly and naturally during the entire stretch.
- Keep your body relaxed during the stretch, avoid tensing your muscles.
- Don't stretch beyond the feeling of slight tension in the muscle being stretched.
- Hold each stretch for a count of at least fifteen seconds.
- Move slowly yet directly from one movement to the next.

Remember, increased flexibility occurs gradually over time, so don't attempt to stretch too far at once. Initially, if you find you cannot hold a particular stretch for the full count of fifteen, this means you are stretching too far. Instead of decreasing the count, decrease the range of the stretch to a point you can hold for the full count of fifteen. Stretching is not a competitive activity; it is merely a means to an end: increased flexibility in the muscles. Increased flexibility is achieved over time through repeated and proper performance of the entire movement.

After you have performed the *Golf Flex* routine for a while, you will find that your muscles are more flexible and that you can more easily stretch to a point that previously gave you difficulty. It is important to continue to increase the range of the stretch as this occurs. This is because the muscles become accustomed to stretching to a particular point and flexibility of the muscles can only be increased by stretching beyond the point to which they have become accustomed. Continued stretching to a point to which the muscles have become accustomed will maintain flexibility to this point but will not serve to increase muscle flexibility beyond this point. Thus, once you reach a point to which you can stretch comfortably, it is important to try continually to stretch a bit farther in order to increase, rather than merely maintain, muscle flexibility and range of motion. Keeping a record of each training program using the Golf Fit Training Log in Appendix C will assist you in monitoring your progress and continually evaluating the difficulty of your stretching program.

For each *Golf Flex* exercise, we have identified the target muscles and the golf advantage to increasing flexibility in these muscles. The starting position of the exercise and the body movement involved in the exercise are described in detail and with photos. We have also listed certain points to focus on when performing the movement, some common mistakes to avoid in performing the movement, and the approximate amount of time it should take to perform the movement.

Golf Flex—List of Exercises

Golf Flex Exercise One: Neck Twists

Golf Flex Exercise Two: Discus (Coil) Twists

Golf Flex Exercise Three: Horizontal Shoulder Stretch

Golf Flex Exercise Four: Vertical Shoulder Stretch

Golf Flex Exercise Five: Chest Stretch

Golf Flex Exercise Six: Seated Butterfly Twists

Golf Flex Exercise Seven: Lying Twists

Golf Flex Exercise Eight: Seated Twists

Golf Flex Exercise Nine: Seated Leg Stretch

Golf Flex Exercise Ten: Leg Pull

Golf Flex Exercise Eleven: Calf Stretch

Golf Flex Exercise Twelve: Wrist and Forearm Stretch

Golf Flex—In Detail

Golf Flex Exercise One: Neck Twists

Target Muscles:

This movement will stretch the muscles in your neck and also stretch and strengthen the muscles of your lower back.

Golf Advantage:

Stretching your neck muscles will enable you to rotate your head through a greater range of motion and minimize the risk of injury to your head and neck during the golf swing.

Stretching and strengthening the muscles of your lower back will enable you to rotate your upper body through a greater range of motion, minimize the risk of injury to your lower back, and make it easier and more comfortable to bend and maintain a proper position at address.

Starting Position:

Standing straight, feet shoulder-width apart, knees slightly bent, and toes pointed slightly outward. Bend slightly at the waist, about one third of the way toward being parallel to the floor. Place your hands on your hips or thighs for support. (See Step 1.)

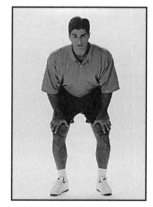

STEP 1

Description of Movement:

Keeping your back straight and without moving your upper torso or shoulders, look over your right shoulder by rotating your head to the right until you feel a slight pull

49

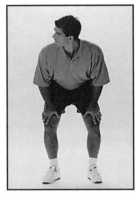

STEP 2

in the left side of your neck. (See Step 2.) Pause and hold your head in this position for a full count of fifteen. Slowly look over your left shoulder by rotating your head to the left until you feel a slight pull in the right side of your neck. Pause and hold your head in this position for a full count of fifteen.

Focus On:

Maintaining the slight tension in the side of your neck for the full count of fifteen.

Keeping your back straight.

Keeping your shoulders facing forward.

Common Mistakes to Avoid:

Arching your back.

Turning your shoulders or upper body.

Tilting your head forward or backward.

Rotating your head too quickly or beyond the slight tension in the side of your neck

Approximate Time: 45 seconds.

Golf Flex Exercise Two: Discus (Coil) Stretch

Target Muscles:

This exercise will stretch all the muscle groups involved in rotating the trunk during the golf swing, which include your shoulders, chest, upper and lower back, abdominals, hips, and upper legs.

Golf Advantage:

Stretching these muscles will enable you to achieve greater overall trunk rotation throughout the golf swing, resulting in decreased risk of injury, greater swing speed, and a more powerful and efficient golf swing.

Starting Position:

Standing straight, feet shoulder-width apart, knees slightly bent, and toes pointed slightly outward. Bend slightly at the waist, about one third of the way toward being parallel to the floor. Extend your arms down straight in front of you, palms facing in. (See Step 1.)

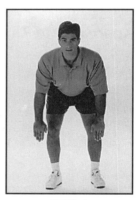

STEP 1

Description of Movement:

Keeping both feet flat on the floor, slowly twist your upper body to the right as far as you comfortably can by moving your left arm in front of your body and toward your right shoulder and your right arm behind your body and back toward your left shoulder. (See Step 2.) You should feel a slight tension in your right side. Pause at the end of the twist and hold this position for a count of fifteen. Slowly return to the

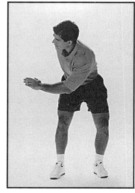

STEP 2

51

original starting position. Perform the same movement to the left side.

Focus On:

Maintaining the slight tension in your side for the full count of fifteen.

Common Mistakes to Avoid:

Raising your heels off the floor.

Arching your back or rounding your shoulders.

Tilting your upper body forward or backward.

Rotating your upper body beyond the feeling of slight tension.

Approximate Time: 45 seconds.

Golf Flex Exercise Three: Horizontal Shoulder Stretch

Target Muscles:

This exercise will stretch the muscles located in your rear shoulder and upper back.

Golf Advantage:

Stretching the muscles of your rear shoulder and upper back will enable you to rotate your shoulders through a greater range of motion during the golf swing, minimize the risk of injury to these muscles, and enable you to generate greater swing speed.

Starting Position:

Standing straight, feet shoulder-width apart, knees slightly bent, and toes pointed slightly outward.

Description of Movement:

Bend your right arm about ninety degrees, and slowly extend it forward so that your right elbow moves toward the middle of your body and your right hand is reaching toward your left shoulder. Place your left hand behind your right elbow, and pull your right elbow toward your left shoulder until you feel a slight tension in your right shoulder. Allow your right hand to move over your left shoulder. (See Step 1.) Hold this position for a count of fifteen. Slowly release your right elbow and return to the starting position. Perform the same movement with the left arm.

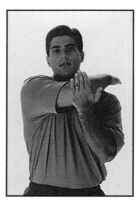

STEP 1

Focus On:

Maintaining the slight tension in your shoulder for the full count of fifteen.

Keeping the extended arm parallel to the floor.

Common Mistakes to Avoid:

Dropping the elbow of your extended arm below shoulder level.

Pulling the elbow of the extended arm too quickly or beyond the point where you feel a slight tension in the shoulder.

Approximate Time: 45 seconds.

Golf Flex Exercise Four: Vertical Shoulder Stretch

Target Muscles:

This exercise will stretch the muscles located in the top portion of your shoulder and the tricep muscles located in the back of your upper arm.

Golf Advantage:

Stretching these muscles will increase shoulder rotation and arm extension and enable you to lift and control the golf club better throughout a greater range of motion.

Starting Position:

Standing straight, feet shoulder-width apart, knees slightly bent, and toes pointed slightly outward.

Description of Movement:

Extend your right arm overhead. Bend it so that your right hand falls behind your head. Reach your left hand over your head, and grab your right elbow. Pull your right elbow in toward your head until you feel a slight tension in your right shoulder. Allow your right hand to move down the middle of your back. (See Step 1.) Hold this position for a count of fifteen. Slowly release your right elbow and return to the starting position. Perform the same movement with your left arm.

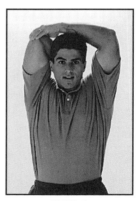

STEP 1

Focus On:

Maintaining the slight tension in your shoulder for the full count of fifteen.

Common Mistakes to Avoid:

Pulling the elbow of the extended arm too quickly or beyond the point where you feel a slight tension in your shoulder.

Approximate Time: 45 seconds.

Golf Flex Exercise Five: Chest Stretch

Target Muscles:
This exercise will stretch your chest muscles.

Golf Advantage:
Stretching your chest muscles will enable you to rotate your trunk and carry your arms throughout a greater range of motion during the golf swing.

Starting Position:
Standing straight, feet shoulder-width apart, knees slightly bent, and toes pointed slightly outward.

Description of Movement:
Extend both arms behind your back and grasp your hands together. Slowly pull your hands up and back while also pulling your shoulders back and pushing your chest outward until you feel a slight tension in your chest. (See Step 1.) Hold this position for a count of fifteen. Slowly relax your shoulders, release your hands, and let your arms fall to the side.

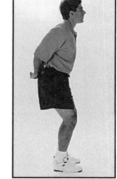

STEP 1

Focus On:
Maintaining the slight tension in the chest for the full count of fifteen.

Common Mistakes to Avoid:
Pulling your hands too far up or back, beyond the feeling of slight tension in the chest.

Leaning your upper body or shoulders forward.

Approximate Time: 30 seconds.

Golf Flex Exercise Six: Seated Butterfly Stretch

Target Muscles:

This exercise will stretch the muscles of your hips, inner thighs, and lower back.

Golf Advantage:

Stretching the muscles of your hips, inner thighs, and lower back will increase the range of motion of these muscles, enabling you to achieve greater hip rotation, and minimize the risk of injury to these muscles.

Starting Position:

Sitting on the floor with your legs bent and the bottoms of your feet touching, head up, back straight, and your hands holding your ankles.

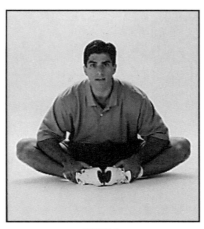

STEP 1

Description of Movement:

Slowly lower your upper body forward toward your legs by bending at the waist. Pull your upper body down until you feel a slight tension in your inner thighs. (See Step 1.) Hold this position for a count of fifteen. Release your ankles and slowly raise your upper body to the starting position.

Focus On:

Maintaining the slight tension in the inner thighs for the full count of fifteen.

Bending at the waist.

Keeping your head up.

Common Mistakes to Avoid:

Arching your back.

Bending at the neck and shoulders.

Approximate Time: 45 seconds.

Golf Flex Exercise Seven: Lying Twists

Target Muscles:

This exercise will stretch the muscles located in your lower back and the sides of your hips.

Golf Advantage:

Stretching these muscles will minimize the risk of lower back and hip injury and enable you to rotate your hips through a greater range of motion throughout the golf swing.

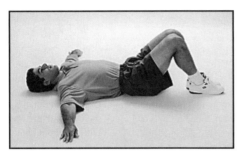

STEP 1

Starting Position:

Lying flat on the floor with your arms outstretched to the sides, legs bent about ninety degrees and the bottoms of your feet touching the floor. (See Step 1.)

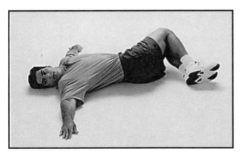

STEP 2

Description of Movement:

Slowly allow your knees to fall to one side. Turn your head to look to the opposite side. (See Step 2.) You should feel a slight tension in your lower back and the side of your hip. Hold this position for a count of fifteen. Slowly raise your legs, and turn your head to the starting position. Perform the same movement to the other side.

Focus On

Allowing your legs to fall to the floor by the force of gravity.

Maintaining the slight tension in your lower back and the side of your hip for the full count of fifteen.

Relaxing your upper body.

Common Mistakes to Avoid:

Forcing your legs to the floor or beyond the slight tension in your lower back and the side of your hips.

Tensing your neck and shoulders.

Approximate Time: 1 minute.

Golf Flex Exercise Eight: Seated Twists

Target Muscles:

This exercise will stretch the muscles of your upper and lower back and the sides of your hips.

Golf Advantage:

Stretching these muscles will minimize the risk of upper and lower back and hip injury and allows you to rotate your trunk and hips through a greater range of motion throughout the golf swing.

Starting Position:

Sit on the floor with your legs straight out in front of you.

Description of Movement:

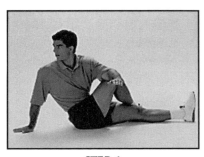

STEP 1

Bend your right leg about ninety degrees, and place your right foot on the floor just to the outside of your left knee. Bend your left arm, and place your left elbow on the outside of your right leg just above the knee. Straighten your right arm, and rest it on the floor behind you for support. Slowly turn your head to look over your right shoulder, and rotate your upper body toward your supporting right arm. (See Step 1.) You should feel a slight tension in your lower back and right hip. Hold this position for a count of fifteen. Slowly relax, and return to the starting position. Perform the same movement to the other side.

Focus On:

Maintaining the slight tension in your lower back and hip for the full count of fifteen.

Common Mistakes to Avoid:

Arching your back.

Tensing your neck and shoulders.

Approximate Time: 1 minute.

Golf Flex Exercise Nine: Seated Leg Stretch

Target Muscles:

This exercise will stretch the hamstring muscles located in the back of your upper leg and the muscles of your lower back.

Golf Advantage:

Stretching these muscles will minimize the risk of lower back injury and enable you to bend more comfortably and safely and maintain a proper position at address.

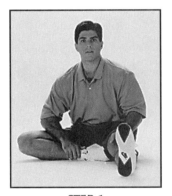

STEP 1

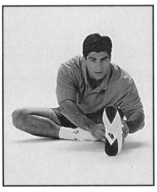

STEP 2

Starting Position:

Sitting on the floor with your legs straight out in front of you. Bend your right leg about ninety degrees, and place the bottom of your right foot along the inside of your left thigh. Your entire right leg should be touching the floor. (See Step 1.)

Description of Movement:

Keeping your back straight and your head up, slowly bend forward at the waist toward your left leg, extending your arms toward your left foot. (See Step 2.) You should feel a slight tension in the back of your left thigh. Hold this position for a count of fifteen. Switch positions, and perform the same movement to the right leg.

Focus On:

Maintaining the slight tension in the back of your leg for the full count of fifteen.

Bending forward at the waist.

Keeping your back straight.

Common Mistakes to Avoid:

Arching your back.

Bending at the neck and shoulders.

Approximate Time: 1 minute.

Golf Flex Exercise Ten: Leg Pull

Target Muscles:

This exercise will stretch the muscles of your lower back and your hamstrings.

Golf Advantage:

Stretching these muscles will minimize the risk of lower back injury and enable you to bend more comfortably and safely and maintain a proper position at address.

Starting Position:

Lying flat on the floor with your arms extended down to your sides. (See Step 1.)

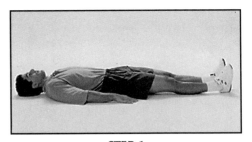

STEP 1

Description of Movement:

Lift your knees toward your chest, and grab the back of your knees with your hands. Slowly pull your knees up and in toward your chest, until you feel a slight tension in your lower back and the sides of your hips. (See Step 2.) Hold this position for a count of fifteen.

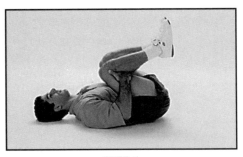

STEP 1

Focus On:

Maintaining the slight tension in your lower back and the sides of your hips for the full count of fifteen.

Keeping your upper body relaxed and on the floor.

Common Mistakes to Avoid:

Tensing your neck and shoulders.

Raising your head off the floor.

Pulling your legs in too quickly or beyond the slight tension in your lower back and the sides of your hips.

Approximate Time: 30 seconds.

Golf Flex Exercise Eleven: Calf Stretch

Target Muscles:
This exercise will stretch the calf muscles located in the back of your lower legs.

Golf Advantage:
Stretching your calf muscles will minimize the risk of injury to these muscles and enable you to achieve greater extension of the lower leg on your backswing and follow-through.

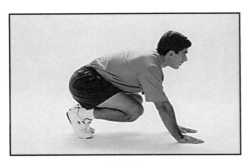

STEP 1

Starting Position:
Squat down on your legs, and place your hands on the floor in front of you for support. (See Step 1.)

Description of Movement:
Extend your right leg back, and raise yourself onto the ball of your right foot until you feel a slight tension in the back of your right lower leg. (See Step 2.) Hold this position for a count of fifteen. Slowly return to the original starting position. Switch legs, and perform the same movement with your left leg.

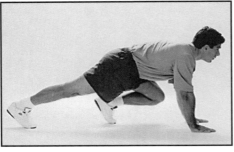

STEP 2

Focus On:

Maintaining the slight tension in the calf muscle of the extended leg for the full count of fifteen.

Common Mistakes to Avoid:

Arching your back or rounding your shoulders.

Approximate Time: 1 minute.

Golf Flex Exercise Twelve: Wrist and Forearm Stretch

Target Muscles:
This exercise will stretch the muscles of your wrists and forearms.

Golf Advantage:
Stretching the muscles of your wrists and forearms will increase their range of motion, minimize risk of injury to these areas, and help you achieve greater club extension on the backswing and follow-through.

Starting Position:
Standing straight, feet shoulder-width apart, knees slightly bent, and toes pointed slightly outward. Bend your right arm about ninety degrees, and extend your right hand out in front of you.

Description of Movement:

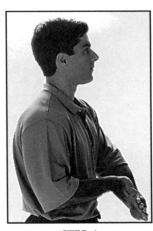
STEP 1

Without moving your right arm, slowly rotate your right hand downward as far as possible so that your right palm is facing up and forward. Place your left hand on your right fingers, and gently push your right hand farther downward until you feel a slight tension in the inside of your right wrist and forearm. (See Step 1.) Hold this position for a count of fifteen. Slowly release your right hand. Without moving your right arm, slowly rotate your right hand up and inward as far as possible so that your right palm is facing in toward your forearm. Place your left hand on the back of your right hand, and gently push your right hand farther inward until you feel a slight tension in the outside of your right wrist and in your forearm. (See Step 2.) Hold this position for a count of fifteen. Slowly release your right hand. Perform the same two movements with your left hand.

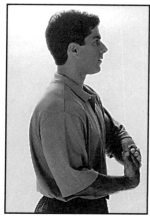

STEP 2

Focus On:

Maintaining the slight tension in your wrist and forearm for the full count of fifteen.

Common Mistakes to Avoid:

Pushing your hand down or inward beyond the feeling of slight tension in your wrist and forearm.

Approximate Time: 1 minute 30 seconds.

CHAPTER 4
Golf Strong–The Golf Fit Strength Training Routine

About *Golf Strong*

In addition to adequate flexibility and range of motion of the golf muscles, a proper, safe, and efficient golf swing requires that you possess the necessary strength in your golf muscles to carry the club throughout the entire swing. Further, golf is a physically demanding activity, and stronger muscles will increase the ability of the muscles to withstand the forces and pressures applied on them throughout the golf swing, minimize the risk of muscle soreness and injury, increase your endurance, and decrease physical and mental fatigue. Stronger golf muscles will also increase the power of your swing, enable you to generate greater swing speed, and improve your control of the golf club.

The *Golf Strong* routine was designed to strengthen *all* the muscles used in the golf swing, as well as other muscles used throughout a round of golf, in the least amount of time. It consists of twelve exercises and should take approximately fifteen minutes to perform. While performing each of the *Golf Strong* exercises, remember to

- Perform the exercise in a slow and controlled manner.

- Perform the exercise through the entire range of motion.

- Breathe naturally, exhaling as you perform the movement and inhaling as you return to the starting position.

- Concentrate on contracting and squeezing the muscle being worked.

- Move slowly yet directly from one exercise to the next.

After you have performed the *Golf Strong* routine for a while, you will find that your muscles are stronger and that you can more easily perform each exercise. When this occurs, it is important to increase the difficulty of the exercise if you wish to continue to increase the strength of the muscles. This is because the muscles become accustomed to working under a particular load and the strength of the muscle can only be further increased by requiring it to work under an increased load. Continued exercising under a load to which the muscles have become accustomed will maintain strength but will not serve to increase the strength of the muscles. Thus, once you can comfortably perform the suggested number of repetitions of a particular exercise, you may wish to increase the level of difficulty of that exercise in order to increase, rather than merely maintain, muscle strength.

The level of difficulty of any particular exercise can be increased in two ways. The easiest way is to focus more intently on the particular muscle being worked, contract the muscle harder during the movement, and hold the contraction for a longer period of time.

The other, and perhaps more traditional, way to increase the difficulty of a particular exercise is to increase the resistance of the movement by using weights in performing the movement. For those who want to increase difficulty in this way, most of the basic *Golf Strong* movements can be performed with the use of hand-held dumbbells. To increase the difficulty of these exercises, we suggest that you add enough weight to make it difficult to perform twelve repetitions, then gradually increase the number of repetitions each time you exercise until you can easily perform fifteen repetitions, at which point you can increase the weight in the same manner, and so on.

For those basic *Golf Strong* exercises that cannot be performed with the use of hand-held dumbbells, we have suggested an alternative method of performing the movement with additional difficulty. In either case, the more difficult, or advanced, method of performing each basic *Golf Strong* exercise is described.

Keeping a record of each training program using the Golf Fit Training Log (Appendix C) will assist you in monitoring your progress, continually evaluating the difficulty of your strength training program, and deciding when and by how much to increase the weight for any particular exercise.

For each *Golf Strong* exercise, we have identified the target muscles and the golf advantage to increasing the strength of these muscles. The starting position of the exercise and the body movement involved in the exercise are described in detail and with photos, and the suggested number of repetitions is listed. An advanced method of performing each exercise is also described. We have also listed certain points to focus on when performing the movement, some common mistakes to avoid in performing the movement, and the approximate amount of time it should take to perform the movement.

Golf Strong—List of Exercises

Golf Strong Exercise One: Lunges

Golf Strong Exercise Two: Lower Back Tri-Set

Golf Strong Exercise Three: Bent-Over Rowing

Golf Strong Exercise Four: Chest Squeeze

Golf Strong Exercise Five: Overhead Presses

Golf Strong Exercise Six: Lateral Raises

Golf Strong Exercise Seven: Shoulder Shrugs

Golf Strong Exercise Eight: Triceps Extensions

Golf Strong Exercise Nine: Biceps Curls

Golf Strong Exercise Ten: Calf Raises

Golf Strong Exercise Eleven: Twisting Abdominal Crunches

Golf Strong Exercise Twelve: Wrist Curls

Golf Strong—In Detail

Golf Strong Exercise One: Lunges

Target Muscles:

This movement will strengthen the muscles of your upper legs, hips, and lower back.

Golf Advantage:

Strengthening the muscles of your upper legs, hips, and lower back will make these muscles better able to withstand the forces applied on them throughout the golf swing, make them less prone to injury, provide greater stability and balance throughout your swing, and enable you to generate greater acceleration and power in your swing.

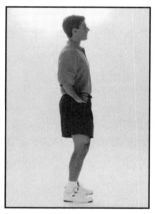

STEP 1

Starting Position:

Standing straight, feet shoulder-width apart, knees slightly bent, and toes pointed slightly outward. Place your hands at your sides or on your hips for support. (See Step 1.)

Description of Movement:

Keeping your back straight and your head up, slowly step forward with your right foot and gently touch your left knee to the floor. (See Step 2.) Pause for a count of one. Slowly push yourself up, and step back with your right leg to the starting position. Slowly step forward with your

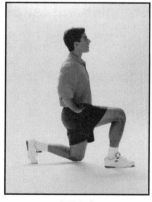

STEP 2

left foot, and gently touch your right knee to the floor. Pause for a count of one. Slowly push yourself up and step back with your left foot to the starting position.

Number of Repetitions:

Try to perform fifteen repetitions with each leg. Bear in mind, however, that this is a difficult exercise to perform, particularly for those who have not exercised regularly in the past. It is important, therefore, to start slowly, perhaps performing less than the suggested fifteen repetitions until you have developed enough strength and coordination in the relevant muscles to perform this exercise for a full fifteen repetitions.

Advanced Method:

Perform the basic movement while holding a weighted dumbbell in each hand.

Focus On:

Stepping forward and back in a slow and controlled manner.

Keeping your head up and looking straight ahead throughout the movement.

Keeping your back straight throughout the movement.

Common Mistakes to Avoid:

Leaning your upper body or head forward during the movement.

Approximate Time: 1 minute 30 seconds.

Golf Strong Exercise Two: Lower Back Tri-Set

Target Muscles:
This movement will strengthen the muscles of your lower back.

Golf Advantage:
These muscles of your lower back are particularly vulnerable to injury. Strengthening these muscles will enable them to better withstand the pressures and strains applied on them throughout the golf swing, making them less prone to injury.

Starting Position:
Kneel down on the floor, and place your hands on the floor in front of you, directly beneath your shoulders, for support. Keep your back straight, head up, and look forward. (See Step 1.)

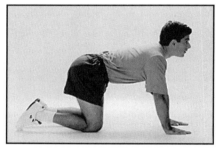

STEP 1

Description of Movement:
This exercise is called a tri-set because it is comprised of three separate exercises for the same muscle group (lower back) performed in succession. For the first movement, slowly arch your back as far up as you comfortably can and at the same time lower your head in toward your chest. (See Step 2.) Pause for a

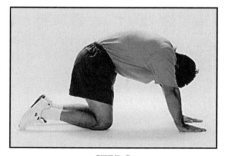

STEP 2

count of one. Relax your back and allow your midsection to sink down toward the floor. (See Step 3.)

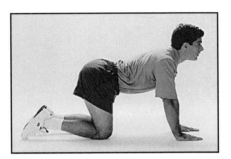

STEP 3

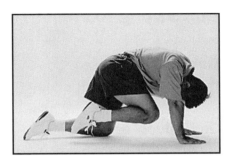

STEP 4

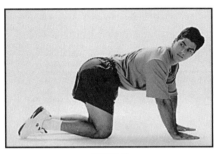

STEP 5

For the second movement, pull your right knee inward and at the same time lower your head in toward your chest. (See Step 4.) Pause for a count of one. Slowly raise your head and extend your leg to return to the starting position. Perform the same movement with your left leg.

For the third movement, slowly rotate your head to the right and look as far back over your right shoulder as you comfortably can. (See Step 5.) Pause for a count of one. Slowly return to the starting position. Slowly rotate your head, and look as far back over your left shoulder as you comfortably can. Slowly return to the starting position.

Number of Repetitions:

Try to perform each of the three movements for fifteen repetitions before moving on to the next movement.

Advanced Method:

Perform the basic movements more slowly and through a greater range of motion, concentrating on your lower back muscles throughout the movements, and hold each pause a bit longer.

Focus On:

Performing each movement in a slow and controlled manner and through the fullest range of motion your body will allow.

Common Mistakes to Avoid:

Performing the movements too quickly or beyond the normal range of motion your body will allow.

Approximate Time: 3 minutes.

Golf Strong Exercise Three: Bent-Over Rowing

Target Muscles:
This movement will strengthen the muscles of your upper back and rear shoulders.

Golf Advantage:
Strengthening the muscles of your upper back and rear shoulders will enable them to better withstand the pressure and strain applied on them during trunk rotation and by the pulling force of the golf club during the swing, making these muscles less prone to injury. Strengthening these muscles will also enable you to add control and power to the arm movements of your golf swing.

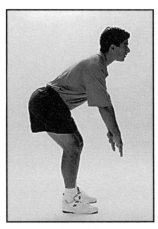

STEP 1

Starting Position:
Standing straight, feet shoulder-width apart, knees slightly bent, and toes pointed slightly outward. Keeping your back straight, bend at the waist as far as you comfortably can, but not lower than parallel to the floor. Extend your arms down straight in front of you, palms facing behind you. (See Step 1.)

Description of Movement:
Keeping your back straight and your elbows in toward your body, slowly pull your elbows up past your upper torso and your hands up even with your upper torso. As you pull your arms up, rotate your hands so that at the top of the movement your palms are facing in toward your body. (See Step 2.) Pause for a count of one, and slowly lower your arms and rotate your hands to the starting position.

Number of Repetitions:

Perform this movement for fifteen repetitions.

Advanced Method:

Perform the basic movement while holding a weighted dumbbell in each hand.

Focus On:

Performing each repetition in a slow and controlled manner.

Keeping your back straight, head up, and upper body still throughout the movement.

STEP 2

Common Mistakes to Avoid:

Arching the back or rounding the shoulders.

Raising your upper body during the movement.

Approximate Time: 1 minute.

Golf Strong Exercise Four: Chest Squeeze

Target Muscles:

This movement will strengthen your chest muscles.

Golf Advantage:

Strengthening your chest muscles will enable you to better control the position of the club in front of your body during the golf swing and will add power to your swing.

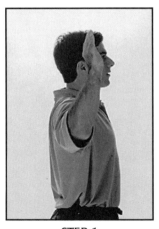

STEP 1

Starting Position:

Standing straight, feet shoulder-width apart, knees slightly bent, and toes pointed slightly outward. Bend your arms ninety degrees, and hold them out to your sides with your upper arms parallel to the floor and your lower arms pointed up. (See Step 1.)

Description of Movement:

Keeping your upper arms at shoulder level and parallel to the floor, slowly rotate your arms in a circular motion out in front of you, trying to touch your elbows along the midpoint of your body. (See Step 2.) Pause for a count of one. Slowly rotate your arms back to the starting position.

Number of Repetitions:

Perform this movement for fifteen repetitions.

Advanced Method:

Perform the basic movement while holding a weighted dumbbell in each hand.

Focus On:

Performing each repetition in a slow and controlled manner.

Contracting and squeezing your chest muscles at the point at which your elbows are touching.

Common Mistakes to Avoid:

Allowing your hands to touch before your elbows do.

Allowing your upper arms to drop below shoulder level.

Approximate Time: 1 minute.

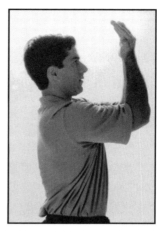

STEP 2

Golf Strong Exercise Five: Overhead Presses

Target Muscles:
This movement will strengthen the muscles in the front shoulder.

Golf Advantage:
Strengthening the muscles of your front shoulder will enable them to better withstand the pressure and strain applied on them during trunk rotation and by the pulling force of the golf club during the swing, making these muscles less prone to injury.

Starting Position:

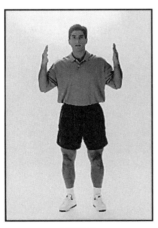

STEP 1

Standing straight, feet shoulder-width apart, knees slightly bent, and toes pointed slightly outward. Bend your arms, and hold your hands up to the side of your shoulders with your palms facing in. (See Step 1.)

Description of Movement:
Slowly extend your arms overhead, and rotate your hands so that at the top portion of the movement your palms are facing forward. (See Step 2.) Pause for a count of one in the fully extended position. Slowly lower your arms, and rotate your hands to the starting position.

Number of Repetitions:
Perform this movement for fifteen repetitions.

Advanced Method:

Perform the basic movement while holding a weighted dumbbell in each hand.

Focus On:

Performing each repetition in a slow and controlled manner.

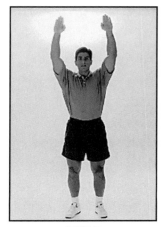

STEP 2

Common Mistakes to Avoid:

Arching your back.

Leaning your upper body forward or backward.

Using your legs to assist in extending your arms.

Moving your arms forward or backward during the movement.

Approximate Time: 1 minute.

Golf Strong Exercise Six: Lateral Raises

Target Muscles:

This movement will strengthen the muscles of your middle and rear shoulder.

Golf Advantage:

Strengthening the muscles of your middle and rear shoulder will enable your shoulder to better withstand the pressure and strain applied on it during trunk rotation and by the pulling force of the golf club during the swing, making your shoulder muscles less prone to injury.

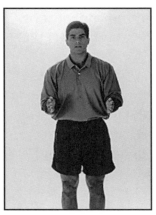

STEP 1

Starting Position:

Standing straight, feet shoulder-width apart, knees slightly bent, and toes pointed slightly outward. Bend your arms ninety degrees, and keep the top of your arms against your upper torso. Your hands should be out in front of you. (See Step 1.)

Description of Movement:

Slowly raise your upper arms out to your sides until they are parallel to the floor. Rotate your hands at the top of the movement so that your palms are facing slightly outward. (See Step 2.) Pause for a count of one. Slowly lower your arms to the starting position.

Number of Repetitions:

Perform this movement for fifteen repetitions.

Advanced Method:

Perform the basic movement while holding a weighted dumbbell in each hand.

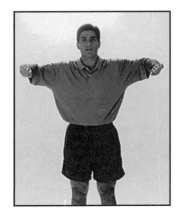

STEP 2

Focus On:

Performing each repetition in a slow and controlled manner.

Keeping your head up and looking forward.

Rotating your hands at the top portion of the movement to feel a slight pressure in your shoulder.

Common Mistakes to Avoid:

Lowering your head or looking down during the movement.

Moving your arms forward during this movement.

Raising your arms above parallel to the floor.

Tensing your neck muscles.

Approximate Time: 1 minute.

Golf Strong Exercise Seven: Shoulder Shrugs

Target Muscles:

This movement will strengthen the muscles in your top shoulder and your neck.

Golf Advantage:

Strengthening the muscles in your top shoulder and your neck will minimize the risk of injury to your head and neck during the golf swing and will better enable your shoulder to withstand the pressure and strain applied on it during trunk rotation and by the pulling force of the golf club during the swing, making the shoulder muscles less prone to injury.

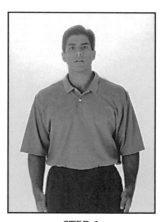

STEP 1

Starting Position:

Standing straight, feet shoulder-width apart, knees slightly bent, and toes pointed slightly outward. Keep your arms extended at your sides with your palms facing in. (See Step 1.)

Description of Movement:

Slowly raise your shoulders up toward your ears. (See Step 2.) Pause for a count of one. Slowly lower your shoulders to the starting position.

Number of Repetitions:

Perform this movement for fifteen repetitions.

Advanced Method:

Perform the basic movement while holding a weighted dumbbell in each hand.

Focus On:

Performing each repetition in a slow and controlled manner.

Keeping your head back and looking forward.

Trying to touch your shoulders to your ears.

Common Mistakes to Avoid:

Lowering your head or looking down during the movement.

Rounding your back.

Leaning your upper body forward.

Approximate Time: 1 minute.

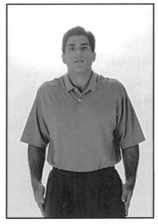

STEP 2

Golf Strong Exercise Eight: Triceps Extensions

Target Muscles:

This movement will strengthen the triceps muscle located in the back portion of your upper arm. The triceps muscle is directly responsible for extending the arm.

Golf Advantage:

Strengthening the triceps muscle will enable you to better control the golf club throughout the golf swing and generate greater club speed at impact.

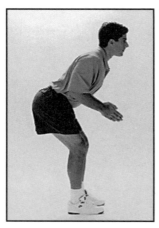

STEP 1

Starting Position:

Standing straight, feet shoulder-width apart, knees slightly bent, and toes pointed slightly outward. Bend at the waist as far as you comfortably can, but not lower than parallel to the floor. Bend your arms ninety degrees, keep your upper arms in, touching your sides. Your hands should be out in front of you. (See Step 1.)

Description of Movement:

Keeping your upper arms still and against your sides, slowly straighten out your arms by extending your hands back behind you while rotating your hands so that your palms are facing slightly behind you at the end of the movement. (See Step 2.) Pause, and hold this position for a count of one. Slowly lower your arms, and rotate your hands back to the starting position.

Number of Repetitions:

Perform this movement for fifteen repetitions.

Advanced Method:

Perform the basic movement while holding a weighted dumbbell in each hand.

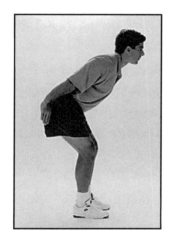

STEP 2

Focus On:

Performing each repetition in a slow and controlled manner.

Keeping your upper body and upper arm still during the movement.

Contracting and squeezing the triceps muscles in the back of your upper arms at the top portion of the movement.

Common Mistakes to Avoid:

Throwing your arm back or using momentum to assist in extending your arm backward.

Extending your arm to the side instead of directly behind you.

Allowing the top portion of your arm to move away from the side of your upper body.

Approximate Time: 1 minute.

Golf Strong Exercise Nine: Biceps Curls

Target Muscles:

This movement will strengthen the biceps muscle located in the front portion of your upper arm. The biceps muscle is directly responsible for pulling in your lower arm and rotating your hand.

Golf Advantage:

Strengthening your biceps muscle will enable you to better control the golf club throughout the golf swing and maintain proper clubhead position throughout the swing.

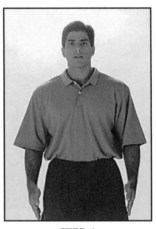
STEP 1

Starting Position:

Standing straight, feet shoulder-width apart, knees slightly bent, and toes pointed slightly outward. Keep your arms extended at your sides, palms facing in toward your body. (See Step 1.)

Description of Movement:

Keeping your upper arms still and against your sides, slowly raise your lower arms up toward your shoulder. While raising your upper arms, slowly rotate your hands up and outward so that at the top of the movement your palms are facing up and slightly outward. (See Step 2.) Pause for a count of one. Slowly lower your arms, and rotate your hands to the starting position.

Number of Repetitions:

Perform this movement for fifteen repetitions.

Advanced Method:

Perform the basic movement while holding a weighted dumbbell in each hand.

Focus On:

Performing each repetition in a slow and controlled manner.

Keeping your upper body and upper arm still during the movement.

Contracting and squeezing the biceps muscles in the front of your upper arms at the top portion of the movement.

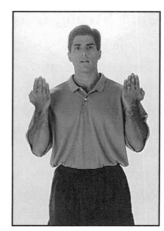

STEP 2

Common Mistakes to Avoid:

Using momentum to assist in raising your arm.

Moving your upper body backward or forward during the movement.

Allowing the top portion of your arm to move away from the side of your upper body.

Keeping your elbows behind your upper body.

Approximate Time: 1 minute.

Golf Strong Exercise Ten: Calf Raises

Target Muscles:

This movement will strengthen the calf muscles, which are located in the back of your lower legs.

Golf Advantage:

Strengthening the calf muscles will enable you to extend your lower legs better and raise yourself up onto the balls of your feet during the golf swing, improve balance throughout the swing, and make your lower leg muscles less prone to injury and soreness.

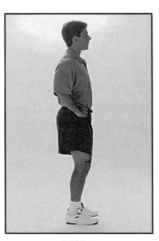

STEP 1

Starting Position:

Standing straight, feet shoulder-width apart, knees slightly bent, and toes pointed slightly outward. Keep your arms relaxed at your sides or on your hips for support. (See Step 1.)

Description of Movement:

Slowly raise yourself up onto the balls of your feet as far as you can. (See Step 2.) Pause for a count of one. Slowly lower yourself to the starting position.

Number of Repetitions:

Perform this movement for fifteen repetitions.

Advanced Method:

Perform the basic movement while holding a weighted dumbbell in each hand.

Focus On:

Performing each repetition in a slow and controlled manner.

Contracting and squeezing the calf muscles at the top of the movement.

Common Mistakes to Avoid:

Using momentum to assist in raising yourself onto the balls of your feet.

Extending your entire leg during the movement.

Leaning your entire body forward during the movement.

Approximate Time: 1 minute.

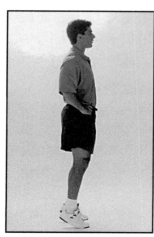

STEP 2

Golf Strong Exercise Eleven: Twisting Abdominal Crunches

Target Muscles:
This movement will strengthen your abdominal muscles.

Golf Advantage:
Strengthening the abdominal muscles will enable you to rotate your trunk more safely and comfortably, provide stability and balance to your lower back throughout the golf swing, making these muscles less prone to injury and soreness, and enable you to maintain proper position at address.

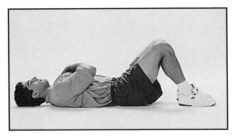
STEP 1

Starting Position:
Lying on the floor with your legs slightly bent and the bottoms of your feet flat on the floor. Hands together resting on your midsection or arms folded across your chest. (See Step 1.)

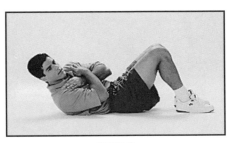
STEP 2

Description of Movement:
Slowly raise your upper body up as far as possible, and rotate your left shoulder toward your right knee. (See Step 2.) Pause for a count of one. Slowly lower your upper body to the floor. Perform the same movement rotating in the opposite direction (i.e., right shoulder to left knee).

Number of Repetitions:

Perform this movement for sixteen repetitions (i.e., eight rotations to the right and eight rotations to the left).

Advanced Method:

Perform the basic movement while holding your hands behind your head. Be careful to avoid the tendency to pull up on your head and shoulders while performing the movement.

Focus On:

Performing each repetition in a slow and controlled manner.

Raising yourself by using the abdominal muscles in the lower torso.

Common Mistakes to Avoid:

Jerking your body up using the muscles in your neck and shoulders.

Tensing the muscles in your neck and shoulders.

Using your legs to assist in raising your body up.

Approximate Time: 1 minute.

Golf Strong Exercise Twelve: Wrist Curls

Target Muscles:

This movement will strengthen the muscles in your wrist and forearm.

Golf Advantage:

Strengthening the muscles of your wrist and forearm will make these muscles better able to withstand the impact of hitting the golf ball, making them less prone to injury, and will enable you to better maintain a proper grip on the club and control the clubhead throughout the golf swing. Strengthening your wrists and forearms will also add power to your tee shot and give you a better feel on short shots.

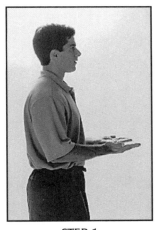

STEP 1

Starting Position:

Standing straight, feet shoulder-width apart, knees slightly bent, and toes pointed slightly outward, bend each arm about ninety degrees and extend each hand and lower arm out in front of you, palms facing up. (See Step 1.)

Description of Movement:

Without moving either arm, slowly extent the fingers of each hand and rotate your hands downward as far as possible so that the palm of each hand is facing up and forward and the fingers are pointing downward. (See Step 2.) Pause, and hold this position for a count of one. Slowly curl the fingers of each hand inward and rotate the hand up and in toward your upper arm as far as possible. (See Step 3.) Pause, and hold this position for a count of one.

Number of Repetitions:

Perform this movement for fifteen repetitions.

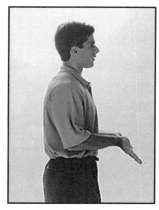

STEP 2

Advanced Method:

Perform the basic movement while holding a weighted dumbbell in each hand. When using dumbbells, you may find it more comfortable to place your lower arms across a chair or table with your hands hanging over the edge.

Focus On:

Performing each repetition in a slow and controlled manner.

Allowing the hands to move throughout the full range of motion, from full extension to full contraction.

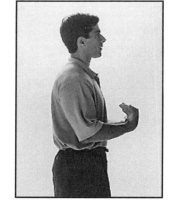

STEP 3

Common Mistakes to Avoid:

Moving your arm to assist in performing the movement.

Rotating your hand to your side during the movement.

Approximate Time: 1 minute.

CHAPTER 5
The Golf Fit Short Routine

About The Golf Fit Short Routine

The Golf Fit Short Routine was developed for individuals who have a very limited amount of time to devote to training their golf muscles but who still wish to increase the strength and flexibility of their golf muscles and experience the benefits offered to golfers by performance training, as well as for those individuals who usually perform either the *Golf Flex* or *Golf Strong* routines but, on a particular day, may have a limited amount of time or simply prefer a shorter workout. It is comprised of six compound movements designed to work all of the major muscle groups using the fewest amount of total exercises and in the absolute shortest amount of time possible. The approximate time needed for performance of each of these exercises is eight minutes.

For each Golf Fit Short Routine exercise, we have described the proper starting position and the movement involved in detail and with photos. We have also listed certain points to focus on when performing the movement and the approximate time it should take to perform the movement.

The Golf Fit Short Routine—List of Exercises

Golf Fit Short Routine Exercise One: Leg Squat

Golf Fit Short Routine Exercise Two: Overhead Press/Toe Raise

Golf Fit Short Routine Exercise Three: Leg Extension/Leg Curl

Golf Fit Short Routine Exercise Four: Lateral Raise/Chest Squeeze

Golf Fit Short Routine Exercise Five: Bent Row/Chest Push-Out

Golf Fit Short Routine Exercise Six: Biceps Curl/Triceps Extension

The Golf Fit Short Routine—In Detail

Golf Fit Short Routine *Exercise One: Leg Squat*

Starting Position:

Standing straight, feet shoulder-width apart, knees slightly bent, and toes pointed slightly outward. Hold your arms across your chest or on your hips for support. (See Step 1.)

Description of Movement:

This exercise is similar to the first exercise of the Golf Fit Warm-Up Routine (i.e., Knee Bends). Slowly lower your body as far as you comfortably can, but in no event lower than parallel to the floor. Keep your heels on the floor throughout the movement. (See Step 2.) Pause at the bottom of the movement. Slowly raise your body to the original starting position. Pause at the top of the movement.

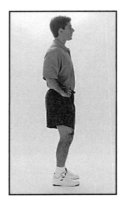
STEP 1

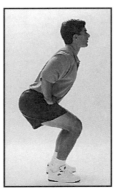
STEP 2

Focus On:

Slowly lowering and raising your body.

Keeping your back straight and head up throughout the entire movement; avoiding leaning forward during the movement.

Keeping your knees and thighs from moving inward during the movement.

Keeping your heels on the floor throughout the movement.

Number of Repetitions:

Perform this movement for twelve repetitions.

Approximate Time: 1 minute 30 seconds.

Golf Fit Short Routine *Exercise Two: Overhead Press/Toe Raise*

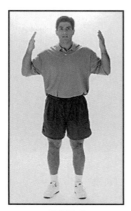

STEP 1

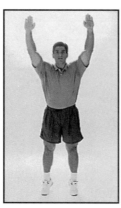

STEP 2

Starting Position:

Standing straight, feet shoulder-width apart, knees slightly bent, and toes pointed slightly outward. Bend your arms, and hold your hands up to the side of your shoulders with your palms facing in. (See Step 1.)

Description of Movement:

Slowly extend your arms overhead, and rotate your hands so that at the top portion of the movement your palms are facing forward. As you raise your arms overhead, slowly raise yourself up onto the balls of your feet. (See Step 2.) Pause for a count of one in the fully extended and raised position. Slowly lower your arms and rotate your hands to the starting position, and lower yourself to the starting position.

Focus On:

Performing each repetition in a slow and controlled manner.

Keeping your upper body vertical throughout the entire movement; avoiding leaning forward or backward.

Number of Repetitions:

Perform this movement for twelve repetitions.

Approximate Time: 1 minute.

Golf Fit Short Routine *Exercise Three: Leg Extension/Leg Curl*

Starting Position:

Standing straight, feet shoulder-width apart, knees slightly bent, and toes pointed slightly outward. Bend your right leg and raise your right foot about twelve inches off the floor. Place your hands on your hips, or hold on to the top of a chair or table with your left hand for support. (See Step 1.)

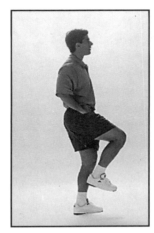

STEP 1

Description of Movement:

Keeping your upper leg still, slowly extend your lower leg forward as far as you comfortably can. (See Step 2.) Pause, and squeeze the muscles in the front of your upper leg. Slowly pull your lower leg back using the muscles in the back of the upper leg. Pause, and squeeze the muscles in the back of your upper leg. (See Step 3.) Perform the same movement with your left leg.

Focus On:

Performing each repetition in a slow and controlled manner.

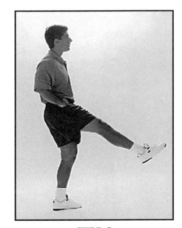

STEP 2

Squeezing the front muscle of your upper leg on extension and the rear muscle of your upper leg on contraction.

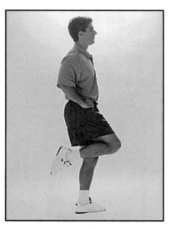

STEP 3

Number of Repetitions:

Perform this movement for twelve repetitions with each leg.

Approximate Time:

1 minute 30 seconds.

Golf Fit Short Routine *Exercise Four: Lateral Raise/Chest Squeeze*

Starting Position:

Standing straight, feet shoulder-width apart, knees slightly bent, and toes pointed slightly outward. Bend your arms ninety degrees and keep the top of your arms against your upper torso. Your hands should be out in front of you. (See Step 1.)

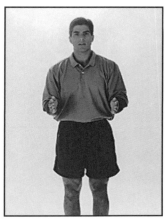

STEP 1

Description of Movement:

Slowly raise your arms out to your sides until your upper arms are parallel to the floor. Rotate your hands at the top of the movement so that your palms are facing slightly outward. (See Step 2.) Pause for a count of one. Keeping your upper arms parallel to the floor, slowly rotate your arms in a circular motion out in front of you, trying to touch your elbows along the midpoint of your body. (See Step 3.) Pause for a count of one. Keeping your upper arms parallel to the floor, slowly rotate your arms back to the side. Pause for a count of one. Slowly lower your arms to the starting position.

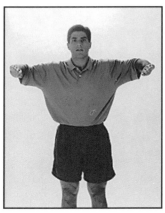

STEP 2

Focus On:

Performing each repetition in a slow and controlled manner.

Keeping your head up and looking forward throughout the entire movement.

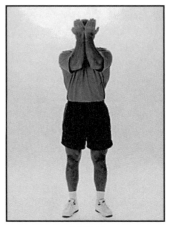

STEP 3

Rotating your hands when your arms are raised to the side to feel a slight pressure in the shoulder and squeezing the muscles in your chest when your elbows are touching in front of you.

Number of Repetitions:

Perform this movement for twelve repetitions.

Approximate Time:

1 minute.

Golf Fit Short Routine *Exercise Five: Bent Row/ Chest Push-Out*

Starting Position:

Standing straight, feet shoulder-width apart, knees slightly bent, and toes pointed slightly outward. Keeping your back straight, bend at the waist as far as you comfortably can, but not lower than parallel to the floor. Extend your arms down straight in front of you, palms facing behind you. (See Step 1.)

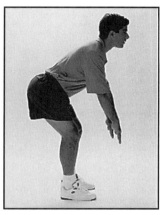

STEP 1

Description of Movement:

Keeping your back straight and your elbows in toward your body, slowly pull your elbows up past your upper torso and your hands up to the side of your chest. As you pull your arms up, rotate your hands so that at the top of the movement your palms are facing in toward your body. (See Step 2.) Pause for a count of one. Keeping your arms in the same position, slowly raise your upper body to the vertical position. Pause for a count of one. Slowly push your hands out in front of you, palms facing forward. (See Step 3.) Pause for a count of one. Slowly pull your arms

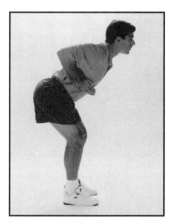

STEP 2

back to your chest, rotating your hands so the palms are facing inward. Pause for a count of one. Slowly bend at the waist, and extend your arms downward, returning to the starting position.

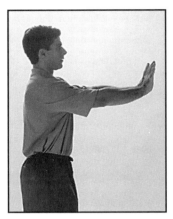

STEP 3

Focus On:

Performing each repetition in a slow and controlled manner.

Keeping your back straight and head up, and bending at the waist; avoid arching your back or bending at the neck and shoulders.

Number of Repetitions:

Perform this movement for twelve repetitions.

Approximate Time:

1 minute 30 seconds.

Golf Fit Short Routine *Exercise Six: Biceps Curl/ Triceps Extension*

Starting Position:

Standing straight, feet shoulder-width apart, knees slightly bent, and toes pointed slightly outward. Keep your arms extended at your sides, palms facing in toward your body. (See Step 1.)

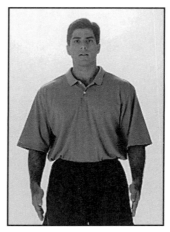

STEP 1

Description of Movement:

Keeping your upper arms still and against your sides, slowly raise your lower arms up toward your shoulder. While raising your lower arms, slowly rotate your hands up and outward so that at the top of the movement your palms are facing back and slightly outward. (See Step 2.) Pause for a count of one, and squeeze the biceps muscle in the front of your upper arm. Slowly extend your lower arms downward, and rotate your hands past the starting position so that in the fully extended position your hands are facing behind you and slightly outward. (See Step 3.) Pause for a count of one, and squeeze the triceps muscle in the back of your upper arm.

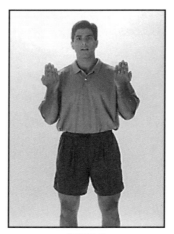

STEP 2

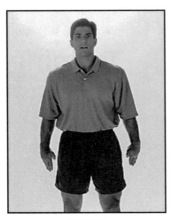

STEP 3

Focus On:

Performing each repetition in a slow and controlled manner.

Keeping the upper body and upper arm still during the movement.

Contracting and squeezing the muscles in the front of your upper arm at the top portion of the movement and in the rear of your upper arm in the fully extended position.

Number of Repetitions:

Perform this movement for twelve repetitions.

Approximate Time: 1 minute.

CHAPTER 6
Aerobic Training

In recent years much emphasis has been placed on aerobic, or cardiovascular, training and fitness. These terms are generally used to describe training and fitness of the heart, lungs, and circulatory systems. The benefits of such training include increased endurance and stamina and lower blood pressure, cholesterol levels, and body fat.

A properly designed aerobic training program, undertaken in addition to the Golf Fit training programs, can improve your endurance, stamina, and overall health, thereby also benefiting your golf play (particularly on later holes). The most efficient way, however, to improve your golf through exercise is to increase the strength and flexibility of your golf muscles by performance of the Golf Fit stretching and strengthening routines presented in this book. We recommend, therefore, that you consider undertaking an aerobic training program only if you have the time and motivation to do so *in addition to* (and not at the expense of) consistent performance of the Golf Fit routines. For those with such time and motivation, there are six components to developing a proper, safe, and effective aerobic program. These are
1. Proper warm-up and cool-down
2. Choosing an appropriate activity to be performed
3. Performing the activity at an appropriate intensity level
4. Performing the activity for an appropriate duration
5. Performing the activity for an appropriate frequency
6. Continued monitoring of the activity level

Each of these components is described briefly below.

1 Proper Warm-up and Cool-Down

A proper warm-up allows the body to gradually prepare for the increase in heart rate, blood pressure, and metabolic rate to be caused by the activity, and a proper cool-down allows the body to gradually return from these increases. A proper warm-up and cool-down are essential to reducing the risk of injury that can result from sudden increases or decreases in physical activity.

The warm-up and cool-down can simply be the performance of the chosen activity in a slow, gradually increasing and decreasing manner for three to five minutes before and after the activity.

2 Choosing an Appropriate Activity to Be Performed

Perhaps the best things about aerobic training are that you can chose from a wide variety of activities and that you can perform different activities on different days depending on personal factors such as interest, motivation, and available time. The activity you choose can be any activity that can sufficiently increase your heart rate to the desired level. Such activities include walking, running, biking, skating, dancing, swimming, and playing tennis. The important thing is to choose an activity (or activities) that you find interesting and enjoyable because this will lead to a greater level of consistency in performing the activity.

Once you've chosen an activity (or activities), it is important to perform it (or them) for an appropriate duration, intensity, and frequency. The guidelines below are general guidelines for achieving maximum aerobic benefit and should be adjusted accordingly based on personal factors such as your current fitness level, motivation, and available time.

3 Performing the Activity at an Appropriate Intensity Level

To achieve maximum aerobic benefit, a chosen activity should be strenuous enough to raise your heart rate to an appropriate level. In other words, if the activity is too easy or too difficult, maximum results will not be achieved or will take longer to achieve.

There are several ways to monitor the level of intensity of a particular activity. The most simple method is to perform the activity at a level of intensity that causes your heart rate and breathing to increase as much as possible but not beyond the point where you can continue to breathe comfortably through your nose or talk.

For those desiring a more technical method of monitoring intensity level, the activity should be performed at a level of intensity that causes your heart rate to increase to at least 60 percent of your maximum heart rate. Your maximum heart rate can be estimated by subtracting your age from 220 (i.e., maximum heart rate = 220—age). Your heart rate during exercise can be measured by taking your pulse for fifteen seconds and multiplying by four.

4 Performing the Activity for an Appropriate Duration

To achieve maximum aerobic results, the activity should be sustained at the desired intensity (i.e., exclusive of warm-up and cool-down) for at least twenty minutes each session.

5 Performing the Activity for an Appropriate Frequency

The activity should initially be performed at least three times each week, with one day's (but no more than two days') rest

117

between any two sessions. After you have reached an initial level of aerobic fitness, you may wish to perform the activity more frequently. Always remember, however, to take at least one or two days off each week to allow your body to rest and recover from the activity.

6 Continued Monitoring of the Activity Level

To achieve maximum aerobic benefits, you should continually monitor your workouts and adjust them as necessary so that they continue to be challenging. This can be done by increasing the intensity of the training session (i.e., by performing the activity in a more strenuous fashion or choosing a more strenuous activity) or the duration of the training session (so that the desired intensity is maintained for a longer period). In addition, try to vary your activity, intensity, and duration to keep the sessions interesting and enjoyable. Remember, the most effective training program is the one you can and will perform regularly.

CHAPTER 7
Proper Nutrition for Better Golf

Many people do not realize that how and what they eat can have a profound impact on their level of physical performance. While it may be foolish to expect golfers to undertake a radical change in their eating habits in the hope of improving their golf game, there is no doubt that a better diet can improve your fitness level, as well as your physical performance in golf or any other activity. To assist you in achieving this, we have provided a few tips on eating before, during, and after a round of golf to increase your physical performance.

Don't arrive at the course hungry or stuffed. Try to eat a reasonable, balanced meal beforehand. The feeling of hunger or extreme fullness is a distraction and can limit physical ability.

Eat during the round. Four hours is a long time to go without eating, especially when you're physically active during that time. If possible, prepare food ahead of time and bring it with you to the course. This will allow you to control what you eat during the round and avoid being a victim of what is available on the snack cart. If you must eat from the snack cart, choose low-fat, high-carbohydrate alternatives, such as pretzels or crackers; choose water or sport drinks over carbonated sodas or alcohol; diet sodas over regular sodas.

Drink plenty of water before, during, and after your round. Adequate water consumption is necessary to prevent dehydration and muscle cramping, which could limit your physical performance. Try to drink at least four to six ounces of water every fifteen minutes, even if you don't feel thirsty. Thirst is a sign that dehydration has already started to occur. Increase the amount of water you drink during extremely hot weather.

Avoid high-sugar foods, such as candy bars and soft drinks. These foods may provide an initial burst of energy, but they will lead to low blood sugar levels and leave you feeling tired and weak.

Avoid consuming alcohol during play. Alcohol consumption can lead to dehydration and fatigue.

Eat reasonably off the course. For optimal physical performance in golf and life, try to maintain a balanced diet consisting of 65 to 70 percent carbohydrates (such as grains, fruits, and vegetables), 15 to 20 percent proteins (with an emphasis on low-fat sources such as chicken, turkey, fish, and lean meats), and 20 to 25 percent fats. Don't get discouraged by dietary setbacks. When you do experience a dietary setback, don't try to overcompensate for it by resorting to a drastic diet. Simply revert back to a reasonable and moderate diet. Avoid fad diets, which at best only provide a short-term, temporary weight loss and, in doing so, can actually do more harm than good.

CHAPTER 8
Fitness of Mind

How many times have we seen a golfer take a magnificent, loose, and fluid practice swing, then step up to the ball, tense up, and take an actual swing that in no way resembles the previous one? Indeed, if we could only swing at the ball as easily as we swing at the blades of grass there would be no need for the myriad of books, coaches, and training devices on the market today. Yet such is not the case. The golf ball, which is only 1.68 inches in diameter and weighs only 1.62 ounces, is capable of producing an amount of fear and intimidation in the minds of otherwise strong men and women that bears no rational relationship to its size.

At first glance, the task of hitting a little ball into a hole almost three times its size appears so simple. Unlike other sports, in golf the golfer takes his shot when he is ready and is not faced with an opponent attempting to block or thwart his efforts. Further, there is ample time between shots to plan and prepare for the next shot. (In a four-hour round of golf, the time spent actually hitting the golf ball is less than *four minutes!*)

Yet it is likely for these reasons that the mind plays such an important role in golf. Unlike other sport participants, the golfer is faced with the task of hitting an immovable object and starting from a stationary position. His actions are not aided by momentum, rhythm, or reaction. He is playing against no one other than himself (and the course), leaving him feeling solely responsible for his success or failure. To make matters worse, he has an eternity between shots to reflect negatively on his prior play and place additional pressure on himself to perform to a certain level on subsequent shots. And each shot is taken under the watchful eye of his playing partners, who may consist of peers, employers, employees, or spouses. Is it any wonder that the mind plays such an important role in the game of golf?

It is unlikely that any movement of the human body has been the subject of such exhaustive scrutiny, analysis, and reanalysis as the golf swing—so much so, in fact, that it is hard to believe that there is anything that can be said about the golf swing that hasn't already been said numerous times before. For this reason, the true breakthroughs in golf instruction will be in the areas of preparation for the sport, both physical and mental. The Golf Fit strength and flexibility training routines will prepare you for the sport's physical demands. Yet a book on golf fitness would not be complete without a discussion of mental fitness and preparation for golf. To assist you in this aspect of your game, we have presented ten tips to better mental fitness for golf.

1 Maintain a Positive Attitude

The importance of maintaining a positive attitude and thinking positive thoughts cannot be overemphasized. A negative attitude will limit your performance as well as your enjoyment of the game. Moreover, negative thoughts have a way of playing themselves out.

Perhaps one of the best examples of a player with a negative attitude is one who, even before his first tee shot, begins negotiating how many mulligans he should be allowed on each hole. (For some of these players, the act of taking their second ball out of their pocket has become so routine it often appears as if it is a part of their follow-through!) Is it any wonder that this player will play below his potential when his expectations are so low even before he begins play?

One sure way to help your golf game is to try to maintain a positive attitude. Think of the game, and particular holes and shots, not as obstacles to be avoided but rather as opportunities to achieve a sense of satisfaction and enjoyment. Phrase any self-instruction in a positive way, such as "aiming toward the left side of the fairway" instead of "away from the water on the right."

2 Be Kind to Yourself

One of the things that surprises me the most about the behavior of many golfers is the way in which they speak to or about themselves during the round. Many golfers wouldn't even consider playing with a partner who spoke to them with even a fraction of the contempt with which they speak to or about themselves. Such negative self-talk is detrimental to your attitude and performance. Try to make it a practice of treating yourself kindly, in a constructive and encouraging manner, or at least with no less respect than you would treat others.

3 Develop and Use Cues

Many golfers find it helpful to develop certain cues to remind them of a key point of their game, such as performing a certain movement in a certain manner. A cue can consist of any word, action, or idea that helps you trigger a desired response. For example, you may adjust your hat before each swing to remind yourself to focus properly or say the word *grip* to remind you to make sure your grip is comfortable before you begin your swing. Experiment with different cues to help you remember and carry out certain key aspects of your game, and develop new cues as your game progresses and different aspects of your game become more important.

4 Develop and Use a Preshot Routine

A preshot routine is a sequence of movements, actions, and thoughts that a player goes through before each shot to prepare himself, both mentally and physically, to hit the shot. All experienced golfers (whether professional or amateur) perform some preshot routine prior to each shot. The purpose of the preshot routine is to provide a time before each shot during which you can gather information and make decisions about the shot, shut out outside distractions, and focus on the physical movements necessary to accomplish the shot. Moreover, by performing the same routine consistently before each shot, the preshot routine provides a sense of consistency and familiarity to each shot, regardless of variables such as where you are playing, with whom, or course conditions.

The aspects of a typical preshot routine may consist of evaluating distance, lie, course obstacles, and other factors effecting the shot, deciding on the appropriate shot and club, taking a deep cleansing breath, visualizing the shot, taking a few practice swings, selecting an intermediate target, and stepping up to and addressing the ball in a particular manner. To be most effective, a preshot routine should not be overly complicated or take too long to perform (i.e., no more than twenty or thirty seconds), should be tailored to your personality and style of play, and should be performed deliberately and consciously before each shot on the course (and every three to five shots on the practice range), whether the shot is a drive, pitch, chip, or putt.

Experiment with different preshot routines to find one which is comfortable and effective for you, and continually monitor and adjust the routine to insure that it maintains its effectiveness.

5 Visualize Your Shots

Many golfers find it helpful to visualize each shot prior to taking the shot. Effective visualization includes visualizing not only the flight of the ball but also the body movements necessary to accomplish the shot. By visualizing each shot beforehand, you are clearly defining the objective of the shot and programming your body to make the desired movements to accomplish this objective.

If you haven't already incorporated visualization into your game, give it a try. Be patient, however. Effective visualization takes practice, and if you have never tried it before it may take a while before you experience results.

6 Narrow Your Focus

Many golfers approach a particular shot with all sorts of thoughts and concerns having nothing at all to do with their proper execution of the shot. They may be concerned with how their partners are playing, whether they will look good on this shot, or the speed of play of the group directly in front of or behind them. Maintaining such a wide focus is distracting and harmful to your game. Before stepping up to the ball, narrow your focus as much as possible so that you are thinking and concerned only about yourself and effectively executing the shot. Thinking about anyone or anything else will take its toll in higher scores.

7 Play in the Present

Many golfers are simply unable to focus their attention fully on the shot they are about to make. Instead, they are thinking about what they did wrong on prior shots or what they must do on subsequent shots. These golfers fail to realize that the most (and only) important shot in golf is the one they are about to hit (although subsequent shots should be considered in determining strategy for the shot). Nothing can be done to cure prior bad shots or to insure proper execution of subsequent shots. Practices such as extrapolating your scores ("If I only birdie the last two holes I'll break ninety for the first time") or worrying about the cause of previous mishits only distract you from properly executing the shot at hand and will adversely effect your overall score.

Focus on playing one shot at a time and playing in the present. Leave your last shot quickly, and don't think about subsequent shots.

8   Set Reasonable Expectations and Goals

It would be foolish for a new golfer to step onto the course and expect (or even hope) to break eighty on his first day or to be a scratch golfer within three months. Most golfers would agree that this novice is setting himself up for a frustrating and disappointing experience and that his longevity in the game is questionable. Yet these same golfers often set expectations and goals for themselves that are beyond a realistic assessment of their own abilities.

In order to be able to set reasonable expectations and goals, it is important to have a realistic assessment of your golfing ability. You should continually assess your ability as objectively as possible and set your expectations and goals accordingly so that they are within reach of your ability. Reasonable expectations and goals will allow you to monitor your improvement and provide a source of satisfaction, motivation, and encouragement. Without reasonable expectations and goals, we cannot improve as golfers and are setting ourselves up for continued frustration and disappointment in the game, as we will continually fail to reach goals that we never had a chance of meeting in the first place.

9   Play Smart Golf

We all know golfers who, faced late in a round with a poor lie in the woods after not hitting a fairway off the tee all day, will pull out a two iron and aim for the pin 180 yards away, carrying water and through a five-foot split in the trees directly ahead. Sound ridiculous? You bet. Yet there is not a golfer among us who cannot empathize with the urge to attempt one of these miracle shots at one time or another during a round. After all, isn't it the one shot like this that we do pull off that keeps us coming back round after round?

Although the one great shot we do make may provide hours of pleasant memories (and boring clubhouse conversation), it is the failed attempts at miracle shots that lead to frustration, poorer shots, horrendous scores on individual holes, and higher overall rounds. Playing good golf requires more than mastering the proper golf swing. It requires playing smart, by exercising patience and self-control and developing and utilizing strategies and tactics that are the most effective for your game.

To play smart golf, you must realize your weaknesses and play conservatively and intelligently at times during the round when you are most vulnerable to these weaknesses. If you are a slow starter, play conservatively and intelligently during the first few holes, building your confidence gradually, until you are comfortable on the course. Likewise, if you are simply having a bad round, or tire easily on later holes, play more conservatively later in the round. Or if a particular aspect of your game is not up to par on a given day, figure out the most effective way to minimize this aspect of your game during the round, such as teeing off with an iron if you've been slicing your drives out of bounds all day.

Playing smart golf requires extreme self-control, but it minimizes frustration and results in lower overall scores.

10 Maintain Your Perspective

The game of golf is just that, a game. As a game, it should provide the golfer with a certain degree of satisfaction and enjoyment. Reminding yourself of these simple truths may help next time you are feeling frustrated and the game seems to have gotten the best of you.

CHAPTER 9
Some Parting Thoughts About *Golf Fit*

I believe that the true benefit offered by *Golf Fit* lies in the fact that it is designed for amateur golfers and offers a variety of time- and energy-efficient exercises and routines that can be tailored to fit within any busy lifestyle. Regardless of your time limitations, there is a *Golf Fit* training program that can be tailored to fit you. Thus, the only thing keeping you from improving your golf game through performance training is your willingness to commit to a performance training program.

When embarking on a program, please remember that the key to the success of any training program is consistency. Avoid any impulse to undertake a program that is too comprehensive for you based on your available time, motivation, and current fitness level. Start slowly with a training program you can and will perform regularly. Then, if you so desire, increase the difficulty of the program to achieve faster results. If, in the course of your training, you experience a decrease in motivation, or if you experience a setback in your training for any other reason (e.g., injury, vacation, or illness), simply return to a program you can perform regularly, or vary your current program to keep it more interesting and progress gradually from there. Setbacks are a part of any successful, long-term training program. Don't let them discourage you from training. You must think of your training as an ongoing part of your normal life, rather than as a program to adopt and later discard after a particular goal is reached.

Perhaps most important, remember that we are each put on this planet for only a short time and we must do our best to squeeze every bit of enjoyment and pleasure into that time. There is more to golf than low scores, defeating an opponent, or winning a tournament. Take the time to enjoy the game, the course, and your fellow golfers. If golf is your pleasure, enjoy it to the fullest. And use *Golf Fit* as a tool to increase the enjoyment you get from golf.

Appendix A. Golf Fit Exercise Chart

The Golf Fit Warm-Up Routine

Exercise One:	Knee Bends
Exercise Two:	Bent Trunk Twists
Exercise Three:	Overhead Side Bends
Exercise Four:	Good Mornings
Exercise Five:	Combination Presses
Exercise Six:	Toe Raises

Golf Flex—The Golf Fit Flexibility Training Routine

Exercise One:	Neck Twists
Exercise Two:	Discus (Coil) Twists
Exercise Three:	Horizontal Shoulder Stretch
Exercise Four:	Vertical Shoulder Stretch
Exercise Five:	Chest Stretch
Exercise Six:	Seated Butterfly Twists
Exercise Seven:	Lying Twists
Exercise Eight:	Seated Twists
Exercise Nine:	Seated Leg Stretch
Exercise Ten:	Leg Pull
Exercise Eleven:	Calf Stretch
Exercise Twelve:	Wrist and Forearm Stretch

Golf Strong—The Golf Fit Strength Training Routine

Exercise One	Lunges
Exercise Two:	Lower Back Tri-Set
Exercise Three:	Bent Over Rowing
Exercise Four:	Chest Squeeze
Exercise Five:	Overhead Presses
Exercise Six:	Lateral Raises
Exercise Seven:	Shoulder Shrugs
Exercise Eight:	Triceps Extensions
Exercise Nine:	Biceps Curls
Exercise Ten:	Calf Raises
Exercise Eleven:	Twisting Abdominal Crunches
Exercise Twelve:	Wrist Curls

The Golf Fit Short Routine

Exercise One:	Leg Squat
Exercise Two:	Overhead Press/Toe Raise
Exercise Three:	Leg Extension/Leg Curl
Exercise Four:	Lateral Raise/Chest Squeeze
Exercise Five:	Bent Row/Chest Push-Out
Exercise Six:	Biceps Curl/Triceps Extension

Appendix B. Golf Fit Warm-Up Chart

Golf Fit Warm-up Routine *Exercise One: Knee Bends*

Standing straight, place a club on your shoulders, behind your neck, and hold on to the club with each hand. Slowly lower your body as far as you comfortably can, but not lower than parallel to the floor. Pause at the bottom of the movement. Slowly raise your body to the original starting position. Pause at the top of the movement. Perform twelve repetitions.

Golf Fit Warm-up Routine *Exercise Two: Bent Trunk Twists*

Standing straight, place a club on your shoulders, behind your neck, and hold on to the club with each hand. Bend slightly at the waist, about one third of the way toward being parallel to the floor. Slowly twist your upper body to one side as far as you comfortably can by moving your right shoulder toward the midpoint of your body. Pause at the end of the twist. Slowly twist your upper body to the opposite side as far as you comfortably can by moving your left shoulder toward the midpoint of your body. Pause at the end of the twist. Perform twelve repetitions.

Golf Fit Warm-up Routine *Exercise Three: Overhead Side Bends*

Standing straight, hold a club with both hands, slightly more than shoulder-width apart, and arms outstretched overhead. Slowly lean your upper body to one side as far as you comfortably can. Pause. Slowly return to the starting position. Pause. Slowly lean your upper body to the opposite side as far as you comfortably can. Pause. Slowly return to the starting position. Perform six repetitions.

Golf Fit Warm-up Routine *Exercise Four: Good Mornings*

Standing straight, place a club on your shoulders, behind your neck, and hold on to the club with each hand. Keeping your back straight and head up, slowly bend forward at the waist as far as you comfortably can. Pause. Slowly raise your body to the starting position. Perform six repetitions.

Golf Fit Warm-up Routine *Exercise Five: Combination Presses*

Standing straight, hold a club with both hands, slightly more than shoulder-width apart, and arms extended downward. Slowly pull the club up to your chest. Pause. Slowly extend your arms forward. Pause. Slowly pull your arms back in to your chest. Pause. Slowly extend your arms overhead. Pause. Slowly pull your arms back down to your chest. Pause. Slowly extend your arms forward again. Pause. Slowly pull your arms back in to your chest. Pause. Slowly lower your arms to their original downward position. Perform six repetitions.

Golf Fit Warm-up Routine *Exercise Six: Toe Raises*

Standing straight, hold a club with both hands, slightly more than shoulder-width apart, and arms extended downward. Slowly raise yourself up onto the balls of your feet as far as you comfortably can. Pause. Slowly lower yourself. Perform twelve repetitions.

Appendix C. Golf Fit Training Log

Date:

Day of Week *(circle one):*

Sunday   Monday   Tuesday   Wednesday   Thursday   Friday   Saturday

Time of Day (start):   A.M./P.M. *(circle one)*

Body Weight:

Golf Fit Routine	Exercise	Count of Stretch/ Number of Repetitions (whichever applicable)	Perceived Level of Difficulty (very easy–moderate–very difficult) *(circle one)*				Comments
			1	2	3	4	5
			1	2	3	4	5
			1	2	3	4	5
			1	2	3	4	5
			1	2	3	4	5
			1	2	3	4	5
			1	2	3	4	5
			1	2	3	4	5
			1	2	3	4	5
			1	2	3	4	5
			1	2	3	4	5
			1	2	3	4	5
			1	2	3	4	5
			1	2	3	4	5
			1	2	3	4	5
			1	2	3	4	5
			1	2	3	4	5
			1	2	3	4	5
			1	2	3	4	5

Time of Day (finish):   A.M./P.M. *(circle one)*

Overall Perceived Level of Program Difficulty: 1   2   3   4   5   6   7   8   9   10
(very easy–moderate–very difficult)

Comments:

Sample Golf Fit Training Log

Date: *September 24, 1997*

Day of Week *(circle one):*
(Sunday) Monday Tuesday Wednesday Thursday Friday Saturday
Time of Day (start): *9:30* (A.M.)/P.M. *(circle one)*
Body Weight: *195 lbs*

Golf Fit Routine	Exercise	Count of Stretch/ Number of Repetitions (whichever applicable)	Perceived Level of Difficulty (very easy–moderate–very difficult) (circle one)					Comments
Golf Fit Warm-up	*Knee Bends*	*12R*	1	2	3	④	5	*Initial difficulty*
	Bent Trk Twists	*12R*	1	2	3	④	5	*caused by soreness*
	O/H Side Bends	*6R*	1	2	3	④	5	*from golf yesterday*
	Good Mornings	*6R*	1	2	3	④	5	
	Combn Presses	*6R*	1	2	③	4	5	
	Toe Raises	*12R*	1	2	③	4	5	
Golf-Flex	*Neck Twists*	*15S*	1	②	3	4	5	*Usual day-after-*
	Discus Twists	*15S*	1	2	③	4	5	*golf shoulder soreness*
	Horizontal Sh Str	*15S*	1	2	③	4	5	*much less.*
	Vertical Sh Str	*15S*	1	2	③	4	5	
	Chest Stretch	*15S*	1	②	3	4	5	
	Std Butterfly Twist	*15S*	1	2	③	4	5	
	Lying Twists	*15S*	1	2	③	4	5	
	Std Twists	*15S*	1	2	③	4	5	
	Std Leg Str	*15S*	1	2	③	4	5	
	Leg Pull	*15S*	1	②	3	4	5	*L. back feels more*
	Calf Str	*15S*	1	②	3	4	5	*relaxed, less tense.*
	Wrist/Forearm Str	*15S*	1	②	3	4	5	

Time of Day (finish): *9:52* (A.M.)/P.M. *(circle one)*
Overall Perceived Level of Program Difficulty: 1 2 3 4 ⑤ 6 7 8 9 10
(very easy–(moderate)–very difficult)

Comments: *Ate light breakfast about 8:30. Been performing above routine for 3 weeks now. Yesterday golf — noticed slightly improved concentration and less fatigue from holes 12-18. Felt less rushed and hurried. Some muscle soreness today, but definitely less than in the past. In fact, soreness decreased as today's program progressed.*

About the Author

Clay S. Harrow has been involved in strength and flexibility training for over twenty years as a student, participant, and personal trainer. He is president of Sportfit Enterprises Inc., a sport training and research company that, among other things, owns and operates World Gym Fitness Center in West Palm Beach, Florida. He also is certified as a personal trainer by the American Council on Exercise, the largest not-for-profit fitness certifier in the world, and has personally trained numerous individuals seeking to improve their performance in particular sports as well as their overall fitness. Both individually and through Sportfit Enterprises, he has made a commitment to developing and promoting sport-specific performance training for amateur athletes so that they can enjoy the benefits of sport-specific performance training currently enjoyed almost exclusively by professional athletes.

Mr. Harrow lives with his wife, Karen, and their two sons, Chase and Hayden, in West Palm Beach, Florida.